EXPECT MIRACLES

Footprints Series
JANE ERRINGTON, Editor

The life stories of individual women and men who were participants in interesting events help nuance larger historical narratives, at times reinforcing those narratives, at other times contradicting them. The Footprints series introduces extraordinary Canadians, past and present, who have led fascinating and important lives at home and throughout the world.

The series includes primarily original manuscripts but may consider the English-language translation of works that have already appeared in another language. The editor of the series welcomes inquiries from authors. If you are in the process of completing a manuscript that you think might fit into the series, please contact her, care of McGill-Queen's University Press, 1010 Sherbrooke Street West, Suite 1720, Montreal, QC H3A 2R7.

Expect Miracles

Recollections of a Lucky Life

DAVID M. CULVER
with Alan Freeman

McGill-Queen's University Press
Montreal & Kingston · London · Ithaca

© McGill-Queen's University Press 2014

ISBN 978-0-7735-4355-3 (cloth)
ISBN 978-0-7735-9072-4 (ePDF)
ISBN 978-0-7735-9073-1 (ePUB)

Legal deposit second quarter 2014
Bibliothèque nationale du Québec

Printed in Canada on acid-free paper that is 100% ancient forest free
(100% post-consumer recycled), processed chlorine free

McGill-Queen's University Press acknowledges the support of the Canada
Council for the Arts for our publishing program. We also acknowledge the
financial support of the Government of Canada through the Canada Book
Fund for our publishing activities.

Every effort has been made to identify, credit, and obtain publication rights from
copyright holders of illustrations in this book. Notice of any errors or omissions
in this regard will be gratefully received and corrections will be made in any
subsequent editions.

Library and Archives Canada Cataloguing in Publication

Culver, David M., 1924–, author
Expect miracles: recollections of a lucky life / David M. Culver with
Alan Freeman.

(Footprints series; 19)
Issued in print and electronic formats.
ISBN 978-0-7735-4355-3 (bound). – ISBN 978-0-7735-9072-4 (ePDF). –
ISBN 978-0-7735-9073-1 (ePUB)

1. Culver, David M., 1924–. 2. Chief executive officers – Québec (Province) –
Montréal – Biography. 3. Businesspeople – Québec (Province) – Montréal –
Biography. 4. Rio Tinto Alcan Inc – Biography. 5. Success in business –
Québec (Province) – Montréal – Biography. 6. Success – Québec (Province) –
Montréal – Biography. 7. Montréal (Québec) – Biography. I. Freeman,
Alan, 1951–, author II. Title. III. Series: Footprints series; 19

HD9539.A62C84 2014   338.7'669722092   C2014-900686-1
                                                       C2014-900687-X

This book was typeset by Interscript in 11.5/14.5 Minion.

To John M.

To Fern

who taught me that next to Godliness comes Beauty

with thanks for the HBS influence in my life, and the support of CAI in my later life!

David C.

Oct 2014.

Contents

Preface

I am old enough to remember a world where even small events were recorded, and their effects on ordinary lives were set down on paper for posterity. People wrote letters, both for business and personal reasons, thanking a client after a successful meeting, congratulating a colleague on a promotion, or keeping a relative in a distant city up to date on the latest news involving a daughter's studies or an upcoming marriage. Letters were written with care because they were meant to last. So were the diaries that many people wrote daily to map out the meandering course of a human life. In today's instantaneous world of 140 characters or less, where our attention span can be measured in nanoseconds, I am not sure if this kind of attention to the details of our lives will ever again be recorded in a way that will be remembered.

I never possessed the discipline to keep a diary or a journal, unlike my mother Fern, who over a period of six decades, from 1926 to 1986, wrote daily without fail of her activities, the events that she witnessed, and her personal thoughts and emotions. These handwritten diaries, all 48,000 pages of them, have survived and are now housed at Canada's public archives in Ottawa, hopefully to be one day shared with a wider audience. While much is written about the impact of big events on big people, and, although she was in fact the most extraordinary of individuals, my mother's diaries were dedicated to the impact of small events on ordinary people. Perhaps it was the nagging knowledge that my mother had recorded her life in such a consistent and detailed fashion that prompted me to write down some of my keenest memories from a long and, hopefully, productive life that has included more than sixty years in business.

Yet it wasn't my mother but my daughter, Diane, who consistently urged me to write down the stories and anecdotes that I've long enjoyed recounting, perhaps once too often, at family dinners or on long car rides. "Dad, you've got to put these stories down for us and for your grandchildren," she would say time and again. Over the years, I have made some tentative efforts at writing such an account, but it was only when Diane suggested I look for a professional writer that the project began to take shape in earnest. Through Diane, I was introduced to Alan Freeman, a former journalist and foreign correspondent for *The Globe and Mail*, who covered Alcan for *The Wall Street Journal* in the 1980s when I was chief executive. Through a year of extensive interviews and research in my files and at Alcan's archives, we put together an account that I believe captures some of the key people, events, and experiences that have marked my years but, more importantly, the ideas and beliefs that continue to shape my life.

Readers of this memoir may note that it includes very little talk about family and my day-to-day office life. My four children are all in their sixties now or close to it. Michael, Diane, Andrew, and Mark are very different individuals, talented, independent personalities with attractive spouses and promising children. In this day and age, this is no accident. The reason can be found in the strength of character, conscientiousness, and fortitude of my wife Mary throughout our sixty-four years of marriage. It speaks of a strong, no-nonsense mother who made a rewarding job out of motherhood, for which I will forever be grateful.

Helping this writing project at every step of the way was Janice Darrah, my personal assistant for the past thirty years. I hired Janice on the recommendation of Frances Bowen, who began working for me when I got my first real promotion at Alcan in 1956. Frances and I collaborated until she retired from the company and returned to her native England twenty-seven years after we had met. Janice and I are still at work together. Only two business partners over a period of fifty-seven years, and the first one recommended her successor. Quite a record!

I have always treasured optimism as the most valuable of human traits. It is so much more fun to see the positive side of things than to get mired in brooding over what can go wrong. Coupled with that positive outlook has been a belief in happenstance, the sense that the most extraordinary things can happen when you least expect them. This leads me to name this modest effort *Expect Miracles: Recollections of a Lucky Life.*

David M. Culver
Montreal
Autumn 2013

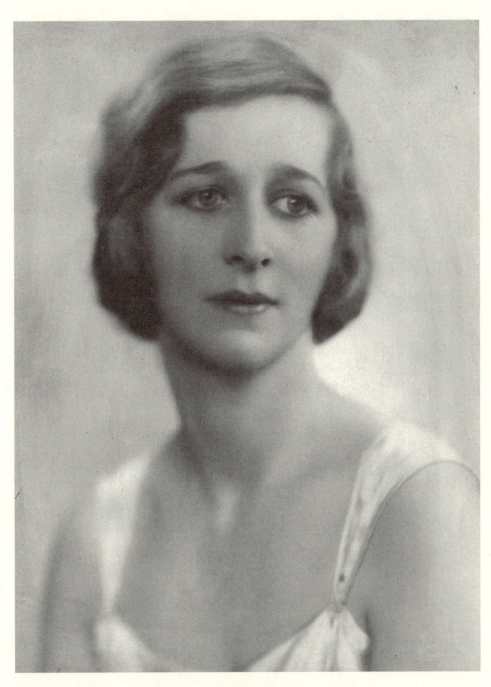

My mother Fern, ca. 1919. Self-educated, grand, and interesting.

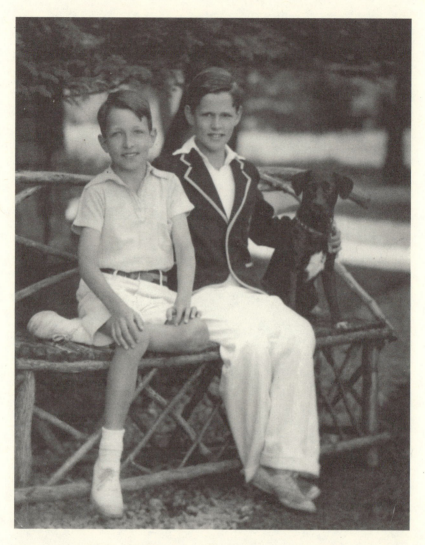

Me at age 9, with brother Bronson in the garden at Murray Bay.

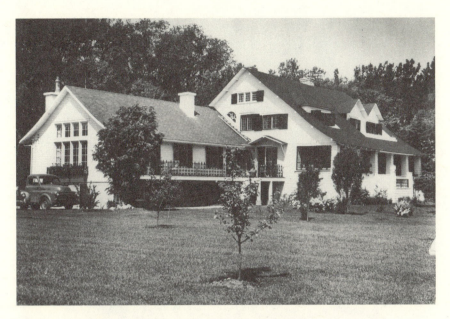

"Blue Cottage" at Murray Bay, built by a granddaughter
of Cornelius Vanderbilt in 1896.

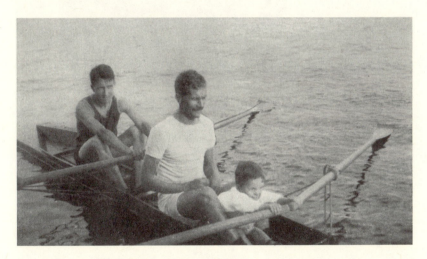

My father Ab with brother-in-law C.S. Riley and his first child Culver in
Winnipeg in 1909. (From Conrad S. Riley, *Rowing Memories*, 1934)

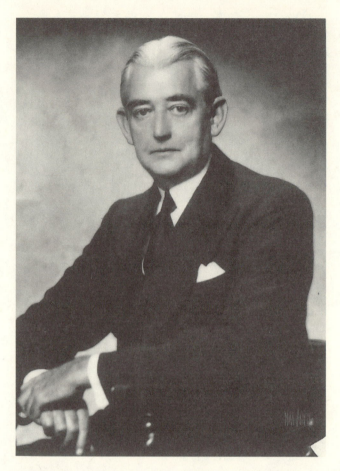

Izaak Walton Killam, little-known Canadian benefactor.
(Courtesy of Killam Trusts)

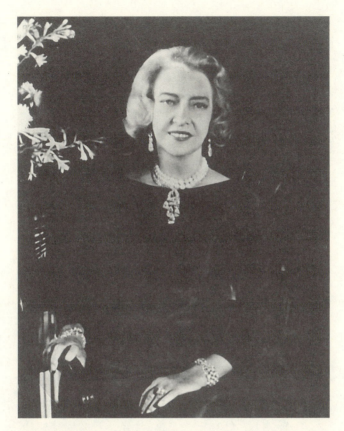

Dorothy Killam, a warm, glamorous, international hostess.
(Courtesy of Killam Trusts)

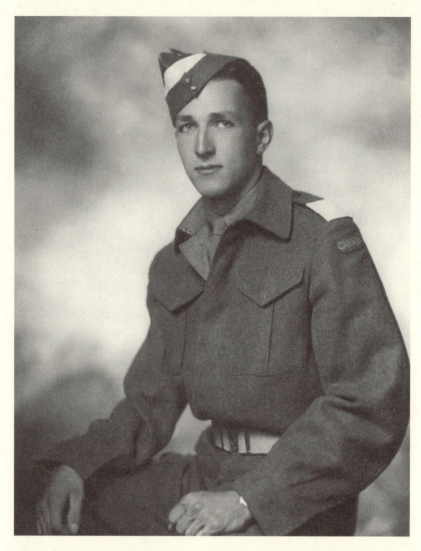

My military career at the Officer Training Camp in Brockville, Ontario.
(Courtesy of Rio Tinto Alcan)

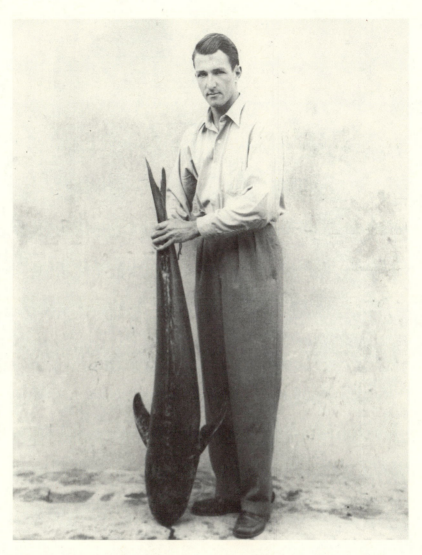

As a guest of Mrs Killam in Nassau, Christmas 1945, I landed a mystery fish.

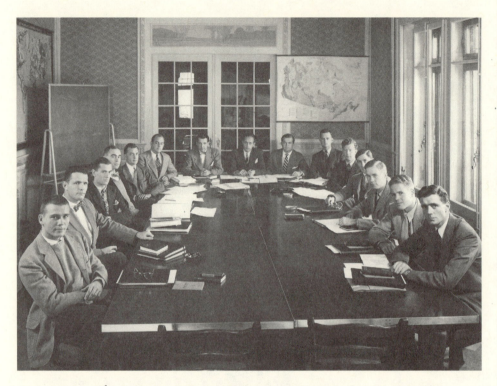

At the Centre d'Études lndustrielles in Geneva, 1950. I'm at the far end of the table wearing a bowtie. (Courtesy of Rio Tinto Alcan)

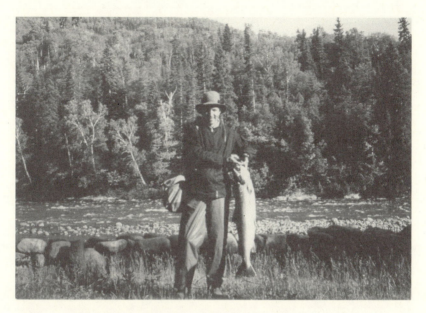

Salmon fishing on the Sainte-Marguerite River, 1960s.

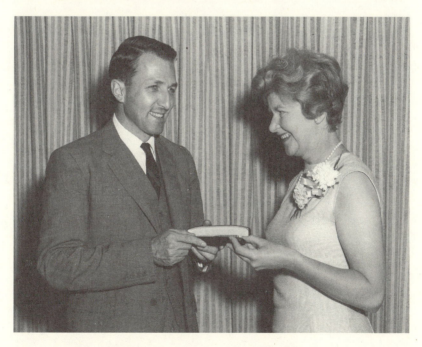

With the indispensable Frances Bowen, perfectionist
and disciplinarian, 1965. (Courtesy of Rio Tinto Alcan)

EXPECT MIRACLES

"Be Emergent!"

Early Memories of Life on a Hill

I had a comfortable, yet uneventful, childhood. Though I was born in Winnipeg, I grew up in Montreal's Golden Square Mile, the downtown area to the west of McGill University and north of Sherbrooke Street that in the nineteenth century had become the enclave of Canada's wealthiest and most powerful families, with names like Molson, Redpath, Van Horne, and McTavish. It was home to the tycoons who built the railways that opened up the West, the strivers and talented businessmen who controlled the banks and industrial empires that shaped modern Canada. With their newfound wealth, they had built themselves grand houses on the slopes of Mount Royal that reflected the scale of their ambition and financial success.

It wasn't what you could really call a neighbourhood, and by the 1920s, when my family settled there, many members of the city's anglophone elite were already migrating westward to Westmount, while wealthy francophones were erecting large homes in Outremont on the other side of the mountain. The stately homes on Sherbrooke Street were being replaced by apartment blocks and hotels like the Ritz-Carlton, and McGill University was starting to encroach on the area as well. Yet despite the hustle and bustle down the hill on Sherbrooke Street, our immediate environment was actually close to bucolic.

In this environment of stately homes, we were actually renters. We lived in Elgin Terrace, a line of twelve row houses at the top of

Peel Street, opposite what is now McGill's Law Faculty. At the
time, Doctor Penfield Avenue had not been cut through, and we
looked out over the Reford property where the owner still kept
horses. I can remember what the rent was on that townhouse. For
a four-storey, twelve-room house with central heating and gar-
dening, the rent was $150 a month. The townhouses have long
since been demolished.

If there was a dominant influence in my early life, it was my
mother, Fern. She was an extraordinary woman, outspoken, independent, and smart. She was largely self-educated, and highly so,
and a great lover of poetry. She could recite poetry by the hour
and always had a poem at the tip of her tongue that seemed to suit
the occasion. Living just across the street from McGill, she would
pop over to the university anytime she heard there was about to be
an interesting lecture although she never formally became a student there.

Perhaps my mother's feistiness and sense of adventure came
from her family's seafaring roots. Her father was of United Empire
Loyalist stock whose ancestors had settled in Halifax to escape
those dastardly American Revolutionaries. Mum used to say that
she didn't know George Washington was supposed to be a hero
until she became an adult. My grandfather, Howard Smith, was a
ship's captain. When he was twenty-one, he inherited a sailing
vessel from his father. It was the late nineteenth century, and the
Smiths sailed that ship once a year from Halifax to Kobe, Japan
and back. The return trip took nine months. The ship took salt fish
from the Maritimes to Japan and brought back silks and other
products, and my grandfather earned enough from that trade to
provide him with a fairly comfortable living.

It was before the days of the Panama Canal so Grandfather
Smith would sail across the Atlantic, down around the tip of
Africa, across the Indian Ocean, and up to Japan. On his first trip
to Japan as a captain, his last port of call before crossing the
Atlantic Ocean for home was Galway in the west of Ireland. Being
twenty-two and feeling his oats, he spied a girl whose looks
appealed to him. He went to her family and asked permission

to marry. Her name was Elizabeth Anne Lynch, a striking, tall woman with black, curly hair and eyes that were described as looking like "pansies under running water." When Elizabeth's parents asked the young captain his religion, he replied simply that he was not a Catholic. So they refused to give their permission for this ecumenical union. Undeterred, my grandfather tucked young Elizabeth under his arm and sailed away to Canada. Today it would be called kidnapping and an arrest warrant would be sent out through Interpol, but in those days it was called high romance. They returned to Halifax, married, and had four children, including Fern who was the third of the brood.

After the fourth child was born, my grandfather said he'd had enough of sailing alone to Asia so he convinced my grandmother to join him on his next voyage. While in Japan, like any other man would have done, he bought his wife a kimono. On their return to Halifax, she decided to dress in the kimono, surely a novelty in Canada at the turn of the twentieth century, to impress her four small children. As she turned around to look at herself in the mirror, the tail of the kimono hit a gaslight and caught fire. My grandmother was burned to death. Fern was just four.

My mother would later tell the story of how she and her siblings surrounded their father to share their grief and plead with him, "Daddy, you must never marry again." His answer to them was categorical. "I will never marry again if you promise me that you will never set foot in Ireland." The fact that he had been refused permission to marry the love of his life was something he could never tolerate or overcome. These were passions of a kind we cannot fathom now.

My grandfather never did remarry. As for Fern, she would attend Baptist Sunday School every week, but, the same afternoon, she would also head off to the Convent of the Sacred Heart for some Catholic instruction, fulfilling a promise made by her father to her mother. One Sunday, my grandfather asked Fern whether she was happy. She replied, admonishing her father, "No, I am not happy. I can't be happy when you do not know that the Catholic faith is the only true faith." Not the kind of message my grandfather wanted to hear, so according to my mother it was the last time she ever set foot in that Convent.

My mother was then sent to Toronto to board at Havergal College, a girls' school that was decidedly Protestant – Church of England to be precise. At fifteen, it was off to London, England to attend a finishing school, known as Ivy House, designed to produce ladies to marry gentlemen. Her father presented Fern to the headmistress and told her, "Now you mustn't teach my daughter mathematics, as it gives her a headache." It was 1912.

The First World War soon intervened, marooning Fern in London. The war cost the life of her brother Bronson, a captain in the Royal Flying Corps, who was shot down by a German flying ace at the age of 22. Then her sister, who was living in Britain, died in childbirth. But that awful war also allowed Fern to meet my father, a lieutenant-colonel in the Canadian Army, whom she met while he was on leave from the front in France. Albert Ferguson Culver was slender, handsome, and quite the sportsman, an accomplished horse jumper, hockey player, and rower, in addition to being a war hero.

The Culvers had arrived in America shortly after the Mayflower and settled in Connecticut. The name was originally spelled as "Colver" but mutated over time to Culver. Family lore says that at one point there were seven brothers, and when the American Revolution came, one of them became a United Empire Loyalist and moved up to Cobourg, Ontario. My Culver forebears lived in Ontario until the late nineteenth century when my grandfather, William Henry Culver, left his law practice in London, Ontario and headed west to Manitoba, seeking his fortune in the great land boom of the era. Admitted to the Manitoba Bar, he was a partner with James A. Aikins in forming the law firm of Aikins, Culver & Hamilton whose successor firm remains Manitoba's oldest and largest law firm.

A good student, my dad attended the University of Manitoba, but it was as an oarsman with the Winnipeg Rowing Club that Ab Culver, or Snapper as he was known to friends, made his mark. The Club was a force to be reckoned with during that period both in Canada and abroad, travelling widely and winning the Steward's Cup at the Henley Regatta in England in 1910. Two years later, my dad was a standout for the Winnipeg Rowing Club at the National Association of Amateur Oarsmen Regatta in Peoria, Illinois where he won the single scull event. Among the vanquished at that event was none other than John B. Kelly of Philadelphia, father of the actress Grace Kelly, who went on to become a triple Olympic gold medal winner.

C. S. Riley, president of the Winnipeg Rowing Club no fewer than seventeen times and my dad's brother-in-law – he had married Jean Culver – was unstinting in his praise of Snapper's rowing prowess. In a memoir published many years later, Con Riley says this about my father: "For his weight, Ab was without doubt one of the fastest scullers that ever sat in a boat."

Like others of his generation, my dad signed up enthusiastically for the Great War, and in March of 1915 he joined the 19th Battery of the Canadian Field Artillery. His sign-up documents describe him as a twenty-five-year-old "gentleman" working for Northern Trust Co., weighing 135 pounds, measuring 5 foot 8.5 inches tall and having a "fresh" complexion. Deployed to France, in 1917 he was awarded the Military Cross for distinguished service in the field, leaving the service with the rank of major. Like so many of that generation who fought in the trenches, he was a victim of the Spanish flu epidemic in early 1919 but was lucky enough to survive.

I'm sure that as a war hero and athlete, Dad cut quite a striking figure. But, Fern had been expected to marry a fellow from her days in Halifax. Sanford Critchley went on to become an officer in the Royal Navy, but Fern found him boring, met my father, and moved on. Yet she never forgot Critchley and kept a picture of him in our house for the rest of her life. My father, not a jealous man and never lacking self-confidence, didn't seem to mind seeing his onetime rival hanging around the house.

As for Critchley, he married and eventually retired to New Zealand. In the late 1970s or early 1980s, I was in New Zealand for a meeting of the Pacific Basin Economic Council. On the second or third day, there was a big black-tie dinner party put on by the local people for all these visitors. And at the dinner I was talking to a lady from Christchurch and I asked her whether she had ever heard of an Admiral Critchley. She turned to her husband and said, "Admiral Critchley. We know him, don't we?" Her husband replied, "Well, I don't think he ever made admiral, but he might have been a captain. Yes, we know him. He lives up in Blenheim." On our last day in New Zealand, just before leaving for the airport, I got on the phone and called Critchley. "Hello," he answered in a very deep British voice. I introduced myself. "Admiral Critchley? I'm David Culver from Montreal." "Who?" he replied. "I'm the second son of Fern Elizabeth Smith of Halifax." "Good God!" he exclaimed, "My very first love. I still carry a picture of her in my wallet." He regretted not being able to see us during our visit, adding, "Please tell her that I'm still sailing my boat, and I have a little trouble with my knee, but other than that I'm fine." At the time, he must have been well into his eighties.

I came back to Montreal but forgot to mention that call to my mother for quite a while. Then one day I said to her, "By the way, I spoke to Admiral Critchley when I was in New Zealand." She didn't seem to want to talk about it. I dropped the subject, and a couple of weeks later I mentioned it again and said to her, "You didn't seem very interested in my conversation with the admiral." Then she said, "He died last month." It had been more than sixty years but clearly my mother had never forgotten.

My parents were married in Toronto in 1920 and headed back to Dad's hometown, Winnipeg, where he began working in the insurance business. Life on the Canadian prairies was quite a shock for my now-worldly mother. After London and champagne, she discovered that Winnipeg was all Christian Science and Ovaltine. The Rileys, the prominent family into which my Aunt Jean had married, were followers of that faith. Fern loved her extended family but found life on the prairies, with no more evenings of ballet with Nijinsky or concerts featuring Caruso, dull and a bit bleak, so she encouraged my dad to look elsewhere to pursue his career. Aunt Jean had eight children, one of whom married a man named

George Black. They had two sons, Montegu and Conrad, meaning that Conrad Black, the onetime newspaper publisher, is a cousin of mine. During the years when Conrad Black lived in Quebec, he never missed showing up for a Culver family event. His incomparable intellect and knowledge of history and matters cultural made him a favourite of my mother. While I have never contacted him during his recent travails, I have always been proud to call him my first cousin, once removed. His mother, Betty, was the daughter of my father's sister. I vaguely remember Betty saying to my mother many years ago when Conrad was still young, "What are we ever going to do with Conrad?" Now that he has returned home, I firmly believe that Conrad will continue to contribute to society and should be treated with respect.

My brother was born in 1921 and was named Bronson after my aviator uncle who had died in the war. I came along in 1924. When I was just a few months old, my father got a job working for Izaak Walton Killam at Royal Securities, and we moved to Montreal. Thrilled by the idea of moving to Canada's metropolis, Fern shed few tears.

I.W. Killam was an extraordinary man. A native of Yarmouth, Nova Scotia, where the Killam family had produced generations of sea captains and merchants, young Izaak was an entrepreneur from his teenage years. He began hawking newspapers on street corners but quickly organized the distribution of all out-of-town papers in Yarmouth and hired a gang of boys as his agents. When his father died, sixteen-year-old Izaak became head of the family and began work as an office boy in a Halifax bank. He was soon spotted by the hugely ambitious Max Aitken, who was to become a friend, close collaborator, and business partner. When Aitken moved to Britain and set off on his road to fame and fortune as Lord Beaverbrook, Killam took over Beaverbrook's Canadian business, Royal Securities. It was 1919 and Killam was just thirty-four. His minority partner in the venture was Ward Pitfield, who also became a legend in the Canadian investment industry and the father of Michael Pitfield, one of Pierre Trudeau's wisest advisers and later a senator. When Pitfield left the firm in 1927, Killam brought in Herbert Symington, a Winnipeg lawyer, as vice president. Together with my dad, they formed the nucleus of Royal Securities in its heyday, a group dubbed by some wags as The Trinity.

Killam had an approach to investment banking that I would certainly love to emulate, even today. Royal Securities would not take a company public unless Killam was willing to keep forty per cent of the stock himself. In other words, he was putting his money where he was asking other people to put their money. Then he created a great sales force across Canada to spread the other sixty per cent around widely so that no one could effectively challenge what he was doing with the company. Royal Securities was involved in a range of industries including electric utilities and pulp and paper companies across Canada and abroad, particularly in Latin America. At one point, Killam was considered the wealthiest man in the country. This all involved heavy borrowing on his part – so heavy that the banks dared not call in their loans during the Depression.

Killam was more than just my father's boss. He had a major influence on me. He and his wife Dorothy, as outgoing and ostentatious as I.W. was quiet and introverted, had no children. They lived in a lovely old limestone house on the corner of Stanley and Sherbrooke Streets in Montreal, which was unfortunately later torn down. Mister Killam, as I called him, was a quiet, very private man. His wife would be away from Montreal a lot, entertaining in England, France, or the Bahamas, so he was often alone at home. Occasionally, he would call up in the evenings and ask me to come down to his house, which was down the hill from Elgin Terrace, to keep him company and do my homework.

I can still remember one spring evening when I was fifteen. We were in the large second-floor study when Mr Killam, sitting in the far corner under a single lightbulb, spoke up, "Young man, never do the wrong thing for the right tax reason." Mr Killam was a number cruncher and not much of a talker. After what seemed to me an endless silence, he continued, "Do you know how much tax I will have to pay when I die?" "No sir," I replied. More silence, then, "I don't have to pay any taxes you know – I own two houses in Nassau," explaining that he could escape the taxman in Canada by becoming a nonresident. More silence. Then he added, "I made the money in Canada; I will pay the tax in Canada." (He was of course referring to the estate taxes that were levied at the time.) Another round of silence and then he said, "I could delay payment by creating a trust, but that would tie Dorothy's hands. Best to pay up, so the day after I go she will be free to do what she pleases with the residue." More silence, then the moral of the tale repeated. "Young man, never do the wrong thing for the right tax reason."

I have never forgotten that admonition. I think I respected it throughout my days at Alcan and since. It has never let me down.

Mr Killam died in 1955. The inheritance taxes paid on his estate totalled some $50 million, a huge sum at the time. The proceeds were used by the Canadian government, along with a similar amount from the estate of Sir James Dunn, to provide the initial funding for the Canada Council for the Arts. Four or five years after Mr Killam died, I was walking up Fifth Avenue in New York when I ran into an absolutely bubbling Dorothy Killam. She gave me a big hug and exclaimed, "David, this is a great day – I've made it all back!" "Made what back?" I wondered. "The tax that Izaak paid. That's what I've made back." "Congratulations – how did you do it?" I asked. "Shortly after I lost him, all the little men in grey suits and fedoras buzzed around me saying that, to be safe, I should diversify. I didn't like the sound of that, so I took a plunge and put all the residue into one stock." "Which stock?" I asked. "A company called I B M ."

Today, when I visit the Montreal Neurological Institute and meet the "Killam Professor" of this and that and read of the many scientific areas supported by the Killam Trusts across Canada, I give thanks for Dorothy Killam's risk taking and for Izaak Walton Killam's decision to do the right thing for the wrong tax reason.

Mum was definitely the dominant personality at home, constantly on my case and my brother's to study and not take the easy way out. My father's more relaxed nature was a welcome foil to her sometimes-bombastic ways. Corporal punishment was not his way, though occasionally my mother might give us a whack with a hairbrush if we were misbehaving. Mum would complain that, "the boys are not doing the right thing" and so forth, while we would be hanging over the banister upstairs listening. And we'd hear my father say, "Oh Fern, don't worry about it; the boys will be alright." It got to the point where Bronson and I would say to each other the one thing that we must never do is disappoint our father.

My brother was always a bit aloof and, at least as far as I was concerned, what I would call self-contained. He was more like my father. I ate my meals with Bronson, who was three years older than I, but he didn't seem much interested in his irritating younger brother. Then one summer, when I was about ten and he was about thirteen, I asked if I could go out with him and his friends. Bronson thought about it for a while and then said, "Well, you can come, but you are not allowed to smoke." I guess that was his way of looking out for my interests without showing it too much.

I used to complain to my mother that people were always telling me I looked like my father. We were both tall and lanky. She gave me an answer that was word for word the following: "Well you're damned lucky because motherhood is a matter of fact, but fatherhood is a matter of opinion." That was typical of my mother's earthy remarks about life in general. I may have shared my father's looks, but when it comes to personality, I have more of my mother in me, more of her belief in "happenstance." One of Fern's favourite expressions was the word "emergent." She would always urge me to get out there and be involved. "If you're tempted to do something, do it. Project yourself. Be emergent!"

Although I lived a protected life, it was hard to escape the harsh winds of the Depression that had swept through Canada. It was the early 1930s – I was not even ten – and one day I came downstairs to the living room at Elgin Terrace and saw a fresh copy of the afternoon newspaper, *The Montreal Star*, sitting on the footstool beside my father's chair. The headline screamed, "Price Brothers Crash." I wasn't sure what to think. When my father came home a short time later, I asked him whether anybody had been killed in that crash. He explained to me that the Price family

owned a pulp and paper business in the Saguenay region and it
had gone broke.

Throughout the Depression, I remember my father, attempting
to be optimistic, saying that next year would be better, and then
next year would be better, and so on. I think of it now when people
ask me what I think will happen to the economy in the face of
seemingly overwhelming world financial problems. I keep on
thinking that we waited eight years, well into the 1930s, and nothing happened, so we may be waiting eight years until the great
financial crisis that began in 2008 is over.

World affairs had a way of lapping over my sheltered boyhood in
other ways. We had a janitor who worked for all twelve houses at
Elgin Terrace. He was a big, tall, blond, hairy German who used
to tell me that Germany in the 1930s finally had a good government. He was a Nazi. Other ideologies were also in the air during
the Depression. I remember saying to my father one day, "What's
wrong with the Communist idea of to each according to his need
and from each according to his ability? It sounds pretty reasonable." My father answered, "Well, it is very reasonable, but no
human being will agree on what his need is or what his ability is.
If everybody would agree on what their need is and their ability is,
and act accordingly, it might work."

I enjoyed school, but nobody could accuse me of being an outstanding student. I only began school when I was seven and first
attended Selwyn House, the well-known Montreal private boys'
school, which at that time was located on Redpath Street, a short
walk from my house. We had good masters at the school, so
even without applying myself very hard, I left Selwyn House with
a fairly good education. Although I never had an outstanding
academic record, on graduation I did manage to win the Lucas
Memorial Medal, which was awarded to what could be best
described as the most well rounded student. As the description put
it, the winner was, "the senior student who is deemed by the staff
and his classmates to have made the most outstanding contribu-
tion to the life of the school by way of academic achievement, leadership in games and activities, and by good example."

Selwyn House offered up plenty of sports but never really took them seriously. I can recall them assigning junior masters just off the boat from England to coach hockey when they hardly had a clue which end of a hockey stick to hold. Of course, I participated in everything from soccer and cricket to skiing and what was called "colours," which was basically house-league hockey. I was far from proficient in hockey, but Selwyn House seemed anxious to make me sound a lot better than I was, with the yearbook calling me, "a hard-working forward, a good shot, passed very well and excellent poke checker." Kind words but not very accurate.

Selwyn House only went to Grade 9, following the English tradition where boys of that age went off to boarding school. My family was going to send me to school in Switzerland, but it was 1939 and with war clouds gathering over Europe they decided against it and sent me instead to Lower Canada College, which my brother had attended, in Montreal's West End. Bronson had posed a bit of a problem for LCC because he had led a movement, a rebellion of sorts, to allow the boys to go to the greasy spoon on the corner rather than have lunch at school. So when I arrived, the headmaster, V.C. Wansbrough, who had a bit of a sarcastic streak in him, wondered aloud whether the next Culver was going to be as difficult as the last one.

My English teacher in the tenth grade was none other than Hugh MacLennan, who went on to literary fame as the author of *Two Solitudes* and as one of Canada's most illustrious writers of the era. A native of Nova Scotia, MacLennan had been a Rhodes Scholar at Oxford, but on returning to Canada, times were so tough that he could only find a job teaching high school. His experience at LCC apparently was the inspiration for a segment of *The Watch That Ends the Night*, a novel written by MacLennan after he had moved on to teach at McGill.

He was a good teacher, but I didn't particularly like the course and never paid much attention in class. I was in MacLennan's class on the day in September of 1939 when war was declared and was shocked when he actually burst into tears. It was something that we teenage boys couldn't understand. We all thought that war sounded exciting, and we were actually happy at the prospect of another war in Europe. Hard to believe now.

As for the whole *Two Solitudes* issue, it didn't resonate with me. I knew there were English and French Canadians in Montreal, but I couldn't understand what the fuss was about. I guess that reflects the fact that I was living a pretty protected life.

That same fall of 1939, Mr Wansbrough saw me in the hall and asked whether they were working me too hard or whether I was finding it too easy. He clearly thought it was the latter. At Christmas he announced to me, "This has to stop. I'm going to put you up one class." I was transferred into the matriculation class where you had to write (provincial) exams at the end of the school year. Stupidly, I decided that I would work on the subjects I found interesting and ignore those I didn't. The result: I passed eight out of eleven subjects and failed three.

My mother was furious. She accused me of spending too much time with girls and at parties, so the decision was made to send me to Trinity College School (T C S), a boarding school in Port Hope, Ontario. I didn't mind and quickly discovered that life at boarding school was really quite interesting, I liked the teachers, and the sports were good. The only downside was that they had the English system of fagging, which meant that a new boy was "enslaved" for his first year to one of the senior boys and forced to clean his shoes, make his bed, and things like that. Because I came into the senior class as a new boy, I was given the job of fagging for a boy in a class below me, which was highly unusual. But he ended up being a very nice guy who was in many ways more mature than I was.

The whole fagging thing didn't really bother me. I played the game. I do that sort of thing. I get in a situation and I play the game. But, it bothered the school administration, so at Christmas they took me off fagging and gave me a token job in the library. I liked T C S. One of the good friends I made there was Larry Clarke, who became a distinguished researcher and entrepreneur, the founder of Spar Aerospace, the firm which designed the Canadarm.

I can't say that I ever was an extraordinary student. In fact, it wasn't until much later, when I attended Harvard Business School that I began to excel in my studies. I was usually in the middle of the class. I remember, many years later when I was chairman of the board of Selwyn House, speaking to Robert Speirs when he retired after a long career as headmaster of the school. "You've kept track of every boy that has left Selwyn House," I said. "You know where they all are, what they are doing. Any relationship between the marks that they got at Selwyn House and what happened to them in the future?" He responded, "Watch the boys in the middle of the class. The boys at the bottom of the class are usually there for a reason and the boys at the top found it too easy. It's the boys in the middle who got out of school and didn't find things easy, who went places."

Some of my fondest memories are of our summer holidays. In 1929, my mother, showing her excellent perceptiveness, decided that if she was ever going to take her boys to France it would have to be that summer because it might not happen later. We spent the summer of 1929, just before the awful stock market crash, in Brittany. I was four. Dad came for a few weeks, but we spent most of the summer being looked after by our nanny at a house near the beach. Being by the sea was loads of fun for my brother and me. I still have this clear memory of seeing a big, strong man on the beach, wearing what can only be described as a G-string. He was throwing a boomerang. That image was quite an eye-opener for a small boy from the protected world of the Golden Square Mile who had not yet started school.

As for my mother, she spent a fair bit of time in Paris that summer, visiting museums and buying clothes. She spoke French, very loudly, and with a very English accent, acquired courtesy of Ivy House and which she never lost. Though strictly speaking she may not have been bilingual, Mum never was shy about making herself heard and understood in the language of Molière. Years later, when she was well into her 80s, she returned to Montreal after spending the month of February in Florida only to discover that her Quebec license plate renewal had somehow not been processed even though she had mailed in the fee. With time running out before the plates expired, she had to act quickly.

Unwilling to risk surrendering her right to drive for even a day, she drove up to the Quebec government's central license bureau on Crémazie Boulevard in the city's north end. There was a massive queue outside the office. Refusing to put up with a wait of two or three hours, she forcefully approached the building entrance and was confronted by a security guard. Not missing a beat, she declared in her best finishing school French, "J'ai un rendez-vous avec Monsieur Savard," counting on the probability that there must be somebody in the sprawling office with that relatively common French Canadian name. She was quickly let in. Figuring she had to be a bit more specific if the ruse was going to continue to work, she then told the receptionist, "J'ai un rendez-vous avec Monsieur Jean-Paul Savard." To which the receptionist responded, "Non madame, c'est Jean-Charles Savard." Mum shot back, "Oh oui, je m'excuse, Jean-Charles Savard." The woman responded, "Oui madame, attendez un instant." She was then guided into Mr Savard's office, ahead of the scores of motorists patiently waiting on the sidewalk outside. A few minutes later, she emerged with her shiny new plates.

After that lovely holiday in Brittany, my mother decided that it would be best to stay closer to home for future summer holidays. In June of 1930, we headed to La Malbaie. It was the start of a love affair for Mum that lasted until her death in 1995. Murray Bay, as we called it at the time, sits on the north shore of the St Lawrence, downstream from Quebec City, where the fresh water of the mighty river joins the salt water of the ocean on its way to the Gulf and the Atlantic Ocean.

Starting in the mid-nineteenth century, Murray Bay had developed into a tourist spot for well-off Americans and Canadians who were thrilled to leave the stifling summer weather of the city for the glorious fresh air and spectacular scenery of Charlevoix County. Remember, those were the days before air conditioning when summer in Montreal or Toronto, let alone New York or Boston, could be intolerable.

Summers at Murray Bay were a formative part of my life. In fact, I have clearer childhood memories of Murray Bay than I do of

Montreal. As soon as school ended, we would pile into the family's grey-tinted Hupmobile for the thirteen-hour drive to Murray Bay. If my father was at the wheel, the trip took on the complexion of a proper, businesslike outing. He always left dressed formally, wearing a tie, a waistcoat, and hat. When we'd driven out of town into the countryside, he'd take off his hat and leave it on the seat next to him. When we arrived at the next town, he'd put his hat back on.

When Dad was busy at work and Mother was at the wheel, the journey took on a completely different aspect. There would be unscheduled stops at unscheduled places. Whenever the spirit moved her, Fern would pull over to the side of the road, take out her notebook and begin writing. If she saw a side road that caught her fancy, she'd say, "Let's take this and see where it goes." And if the side road did a loop and ended back at the main road, she'd often exclaim, "Let's do that again." It was a theme Mum would come back to all the time. She used to say that the art of reading is rereading and the art of visiting is revisiting. By contrast, with my father at the wheel, we'd know exactly when we'd arrive in Murray Bay. It was much more of a lottery with my mother in charge.

Dad would also come up to Murray Bay on weekends and for the whole month of August. Like other weekend visitors, he would take a riverboat operated by Canada Steamship Lines that would leave Montreal Friday evening at 7 p.m. and arrive in Murray Bay by noon on Saturday.

In Murray Bay, we rented a house from a descendant of the railway tycoon Cornelius Vanderbilt, who, like other wealthy Americans including the family of President William Howard Taft, owned beautiful homes in the region. The house was called Blue Cottage and formed a trio of homes known as the Yellow, Pink, and Blue Cottages built in the same period at the turn of the twentieth century. Sitting in a dale, it had an unobstructed view of the river before it.

Blue Cottage had been built by Jean-Charles Warren, a master builder and self-taught architect whose brilliant designs and expert workmanship were evident in the sixty villas and public buildings he designed in the region between 1895 and 1925. It was the golden age of summer homes in La Malbaie and the surrounding region.

The cottage, a sprawling affair with several bedrooms, had wonderful china, glass, and silverware. My mother could never understand why the house had been outfitted so beautifully when in fact it was used very little by its owners. Then she learned that Canada's governor general, Lord Byng of Vimy, had used the house for a sojourn in Murray Bay in the summer of 1926 so it obviously needed to be appointed accordingly. Byng's honorary aide-de-camp at the time was none other than Georges Vanier, hero of the First World War and a future governor general, whose father-in-law, Judge Charles Archer, was staying next door at Yellow Cottage, known also as Rayon d'Or. The Vaniers were based at the Citadelle in Quebec City but spent several days a week at Murray Bay, and both Georges and his young wife Pauline frequently took walks along the shore or the nearby boulevard with Lord Byng.

According to an account in *The New Yorker* magazine at the time, Lord Byng's visit was quite the occasion, even outshining the presence of former President Taft. "Mr Taft's ménage cannot compare with General Byng's équipage," the unidentified columnist wrote with dollops of sarcasm. "Canada's ruler is no believer in President Coolidge's theory of travelling in a compartment. He comes to Murray Bay in his private train of six or seven cars with a staff of 26, ranging from his First Secretary to the vice assistant door opener. Train and staff are parked on a siding while he removes to his cottage." Byng had come to Murray Bay in the midst of what came to be known as the King-Byng Affair, a constitutional crisis that pitted Liberal Prime Minister William Mackenzie King against Byng on the explosive issue of who had the right to call an election. Mackenzie King headed a minority government that had been defeated in the House of Commons, and on 26 June he asked Byng to dissolve Parliament so that elections could be held. Byng refused, noting that the Conservatives under Arthur Meighen were in a position to form a government without the need for a new election. Meighen attempted to form a government but was defeated three days later and an election was called, which Mackenzie King eventually won.

We continued to rent Blue Cottage throughout the 1930s and 1940s. Then after the war my parents bought the house from Marion LaBau Browne who had inherited it from her parents. When Ms LaBau Browne died in 2000 at the age of 93 her obituary in *The New York Times* noted that she had been the last surviving great-grandchild of Cornelius Vanderbilt. Blue Cottage now goes by the name Porte Bonheur, chosen by my mother, and even though I later built a family cottage on Lake Manitou in the Laurentians, much closer to Montreal, until only recently I continued visiting Murray Bay for several days every summer.

Summer at Murray Bay was idyllic. The water of the St Lawrence was chilly, to put it mildly, even in midsummer, but we could swim in the saltwater pool at the Manoir Richelieu, the big chateau-style hotel then operated by Canada Steamship Lines. We could walk there in half an hour from the cottage. Those were the days when kids walked everywhere, they weren't driven. La Malbaie is where I learned to play golf and where I got my initiation into the art of fishing. We would go to lakes in the mountains behind Murray Bay that were full of trout.

Summers in Murray Bay were also a kind of immersion in Canadian history. I learned to fish from a descendant of the victorious Scottish soldiers who were left behind in the newly conquered colony after the British defeated the French at the Battle of the Plains of Abraham in 1759. The Brits were too chintzy to take their troops back home so they gave them land instead. The man who taught me to fish was called McLean, but his family hadn't spoken a word of English in five generations. Monsieur McLean lived next to a convenience store – a dépanneur – owned by one Jimmy McNichol, who also didn't speak any English. My mother told me the reason there were so many Scottish names in the area was that the soldiers, when told they weren't going home and were given a choice of land in Quebec, opted to settle around La Malbaie because the light there is the same as in northern

Scotland. To this day, the pure quality of this northern light is why so many artists are attracted to La Malbaie and nearby towns like Baie Saint-Paul.

But in the 1930s Murray Bay was a pocket of affluence in a province that was still largely rural and had yet to benefit from growing urban prosperity. In those days, you would go two miles out of La Malbaie and find yourself in really poor country. There were dirt roads, no paint on the houses, no flower gardens, no cars. The only charm in the countryside was in the little churches, and pretty soon they had to sell off furniture and religious objects to stay alive. In later years, I often said to myself that if I had been Premier of Quebec when Jean Lesage took over in 1960, I would have done exactly what he did. I would have taken money out of Montreal and spent it in the boondocks to pave roads, and build schools and hospitals. And, the investment has been largely successful. The improvement in the quality of life in rural Quebec during my lifetime has been dramatic.

For my mother, Murray Bay was another venue where she could display her talents for entertaining. Blue Cottage, with its wide vistas overlooking the river, was a wonderful place to have social events. There would be dinner parties for twelve to fourteen, but there could be as many as fifty to sixty people for cocktails, when I was often drafted to help serve the food and drinks. My parents' friends included American families like the Cabots of Boston, who have over the years built one of the world's great landscaped gardens at their home in La Malbaie, but also some of the emerging French Canadian families of the day.

It was in Murray Bay that my mother would most often use her French, spoken badly but loudly and with confidence. Her gardener for more than thirty years was Henri Forgues, who ended up being one of Fern's favourite people in the world. She used to tell Monsieur Forgues, "I want you to make me a strong lock and key, and put all my gin and whiskey in that cabinet and lock it up." Forgues would respond, "Oui, madame." Then she'd tell Forgues, "Do you know why I'm doing this?" And he would respond, "Oui, madame, because I take some of it when you are not here." To which Mum would continue, "You're right, Forgues, you take some of it when I'm not here." So the liquor was placed under lock and key. Of course, as Forgues told us later, "I did put it under lock and key, but I have the key."

While my mother could not really cook herself, she was fabulous at training a local cook and maid every summer at Murray Bay. She would teach them how to handle fancy dinner parties, and at the end of the summer she would inevitably invite them to come back with us to Montreal where she could find them a job. They would say yes, but, invariably, after two or three weeks in Montreal, the local Catholic priest from La Malbaie would arrive for a visit and tell them that they couldn't stay in the big city. They had to come home because their parents missed them and needed them. Such was the influence of the local curé in Quebec before the Quiet Revolution.

2

"A Bunch of People Helping One Man Do a Job"

Learning to Manage

In the fall of 1941, at the tender age of sixteen, I entered McGill University with the intention of studying medicine. I'm not sure exactly why. Perhaps it was my parents' friendship with the great doctors who were involved with McGill at the time, men like Dr Wilder Penfield who founded the Montreal Neurological Institute or Dr Jonathan Meakins, an innovative researcher who was Dean of McGill's Faculty of Medicine. They were frequent dinner guests at home and maybe some of their brilliance, or at least their commitment to medicine, had inspired me.

There was a lot going on at the time so my studies weren't necessarily my top priority. I joined a fraternity, Alpha Delta Phi, and spent much of my time at the frat house on McTavish Street next door to McGill's Faculty Club. To be honest, there were a lot of parties. And there was the war and the excitement that seemed to be waiting for me once I turned eighteen and could legally sign up. It's hard to explain now, but my friends and I thought that the idea of joining the army and joining the fight in Europe was unbelievably exciting. So my first eighteen months at McGill were largely a game of waiting until I was old enough to volunteer.

As my second year began, in the fall of 1942, I started counting down the days until my birthday in December of 1942. One Friday I wrote a chemistry exam for a professor named Hatcher and figured out quite quickly that I had probably failed. McGill had a policy of giving students credit for a full academic year if you signed up for the war anytime during the course of the session, but a failing grade in chemistry was sure to wreck those plans and force me to repeat the year when the war ended. The following Monday I parked myself outside Prof. Hatcher's office and waited for him to arrive. He was a short man with a quick, bustling step, and after a few minutes he pranced into his office with a huge bundle of papers under his arm and asked me, "What can I do for you?" I explained that one of the papers he was carrying was surely mine, and I suspected I hadn't done well. I then shamelessly made my pitch. "I'm about to join the army and I'd just as soon not have a failing mark before I go up." Prof. Hatcher cut the string around the sheaf of papers and shuffled through them, pulling out my exam with a grade of 44+ out of 100 scrawled on it. Hatcher looked at me and repeated, "You're joining the army in a few weeks?" I nodded. Then he crossed out the 44+ and changed it to 50+. I had talked my way into full credit for second year.

When my birthday rolled around, I signed up. All of my glamorous friends had either joined the air force or the navy. It seemed to be the thing to do, but I and a few of my pals took a contrary view and decided that we weren't going to take the glory path, opting instead to join the lowly infantry. Call it reverse snobbery or the perverseness of youth, but there was some real logic behind our decision. The infantry was where they needed people. You can't get anywhere in a war unless you occupy the ground. It's not the air force that controls territory, and it's certainly not the navy. It's the infantry. After signing up, we were immediately sent to officer training school in Brockville, Ontario. I had volunteered with several of my best friends. Three or four of them didn't survive the war. They were sent overseas and were killed in action.

My brother Bronson was already in the artillery, which, after all, was where our father had served in the First World War. "Bron" was soon in England where he managed to land himself quite a cushy job. He became the pilot of an Auster, a small spotter plane that directed gunfire on the front lines, which is what every artillery officer wanted to do. When he first thought of applying to train as an Auster pilot, his commanding officer had responded very haughtily, "Culver, my God, everybody is trying to get into that." But Bron applied anyway and was still waiting to hear back when a short time later he travelled into London on weekend leave. At 11 a.m. on the Sunday morning he found himself sitting in the lobby of the Cumberland Hotel. Who should appear coming down the stairs but his commanding officer with a "bimbo" draped on his arm. Holding back a smirk, Bron saluted the officer most respectfully, and lo and behold, the next day he got sent on the pilot course. Such is the way decisions are sometimes made.

As for my war, there was to be no hanging about in the lobbies of posh London hotels. I spent most of the next two-and-a-half years in Brockville, not as an officer trainee but as an instructor training would-be officers. I started off as a private and was soon promoted to what I believed was the worst rank in the army, a lance corporal without pay. I didn't get any more money than a private, but I had one stripe and was supposed to train guys who were becoming officers. Most were older than me and probably brighter as well. But I loved the work. It involved everything from the parade square to physical training. We did a lot of ten-mile marches at night carrying heavy bags, and things like that. There was a lot of spit and polish and smart uniforms. I was always fairly organized dress-wise, so it wasn't hard for me to be organized in a uniform.

Writing home to my mother, as I did quite regularly, I complained about my rank even though I was actually having a good time overall. "As an acting one-stripe, I get all the work, and all the blame," I wrote. "I had as many bawlings out in four months as a private as I've had in one day here. I don't mind blame for what I did, but this racket is continual and on top of it all, they always talk to me as if they were doing me a favour by giving me this job. I told them I joined the infantry and not this racket, and if they had to bawl me out all the time, they could have my stripe right back."

The parade square could be gruelling, with training often starting at 5:30 in the morning and ending at 9:30 at night and only Wednesday evenings free. Occasionally I was designated to train some of the C W A C S, as members of the Canadian Women's Army Corps were known. With men on parade square, the more you put into it the more you got out of them. With women, on the other hand, no matter how much you put into it, you always got the same out of them. You could stand there and scream orders at women at the height of your powers and in your most cracking military voice, and they would move at the same speed as if you just asked them lazily to stand at attention.

You had to be a bit of a ham on the parade square. A bit of bombast didn't hurt. We had a regimental sergeant major, a fellow named Hall, who was a classic. I figure he had vodka with his orange juice for breakfast because he'd turn up on the parade square at seven or eight in the morning quite clearly boozed up. Nevertheless, he was the smartest looking thing you'd ever seen in your life, with all his ribbons, medals, and stuff. He would be the first person that each new batch of officer candidates would see. And, we would get 1,000 of these newbies every month. His speech to them would always be the same. "My name is Regimental Sergeant Hall and my wife's name is Mrs Hall. And I want youz to realize that when you're here, you're nothing but straws on the stream of life and I can pluck youz at will." Translation, you better shape up or else you're out of here.

Like elsewhere throughout my life, I figured out how to get the most out of the situation. If you played the game in the army, it was actually fun. Most army people hate the parade square, but I liked the music, the band, the marching, and the salutes. I liked all that stuff. I also figured out that there was a pretty simple path to getting some time off the base. The way you could get a forty-eight-hour pass for a weekend away from Brockville was to win the ten-mile cross-country race, which was held every Thursday. I got pretty good at coming first in order to get a pass from Friday to Sunday that would allow me to take the train to Montreal. Yet I got tired of being a lance corporal without pay, so one weekend I went to the air force recruiting office in Montreal and tried to switch to the air force. When I returned to Brockville word had got back about my effort. I got a lecture about trying to join the air force, but then they made me a corporal with pay. Then I was made a sergeant. One day, a notice went up announcing that any non-commissioned officer ready to give up his stripes and revert to Private could apply to go overseas. A bunch of us did exactly that and headed to Halifax and, presumably, on to Europe. When I finally got to Halifax, I received an order to go back to Brockville to get officer training myself. I never did get to Europe. That's the way the army works. I ended the war as a lieutenant.

Even though I never did get overseas, I did get to travel a bit in the army, first to Barrie, Ontario and then to Vernon, British Columbia for night training exercises. Then in early 1945, I was named as one of 410 Canadian soldiers being sent to Fort Benning, Georgia to train with the US Army for the invasion of Japan. That summer my father wrote to me, enclosing a letter from the Dean of Arts and Science at McGill that Dad told me might prove useful. I wasn't sure why he had sent it to me. The letter stated that I was a student in good standing and that I would be accepted back at the university upon application. A short time later the first atom bomb was dropped on Hiroshima, Japan surrendered, and a notice went up that if you could prove you would be accepted back at university you would be demobilized quickly. That letter my father had sent proved extremely useful, and by mid-September 1945 I was out of the army and back at McGill.

Though I never saw battle, the army was a great maturing experience for me. I went back to McGill a better student, more focused. The army also taught me what makes organizations successful. There was a war on and there were lots of chances for upward mobility in the military because, unfortunately, people were constantly being killed. When they weren't losing their lives, people were also burning out at the top, so there were always new opportunities. I learned from that experience that it's very hard to run an organization that isn't growing, but if it is and you give people a chance to grow themselves, they won't disappoint. More than anything, the army made me appreciate the value of being a team player. Doing what you were supposed to do, being orderly, being organized. I still believe that we should have two years of compulsory service for young people in this country, with a choice of doing it either in the armed forces or the social services. And you should be sent to another part of Canada to do it. It would greatly expand young people's knowledge of our country, they would meet different people, and they would learn the value of organization, discipline, and teamwork.

Back at McGill, I finally found a professor who interested me. He was an urbane and impressive man named Raymond Boyer who taught chemistry. He was inspirational. Just as I found myself discovering what great fun it could be to study chemistry, the RCMP marched into the classroom in the middle of a lecture by Prof. Boyer and hauled him away. It was the last we ever saw of him. It turns out that Prof. Boyer was an expert in the top secret explosive RDX and an associate of Fred Rose, the Communist Member of Parliament whose spy ring was exposed in 1945 after the defection of Igor Gouzenko, a clerk at the Soviet Embassy in Ottawa. The professor, a member of a wealthy Quebec family, was accused of passing secrets to the Russians and ended up being the Crown's main witness against Rose at his trial in 1946. In the end, Boyer was sentenced to two years in prison and later took on a second career as a social scientist and criminologist.

Happenstance also played a key role in my decision to switch from medicine to business. I was in my final year at McGill and a member of the university squash team. We were scheduled to travel to Boston for a match against Harvard, and I decided to head down to Cambridge a day early. I hadn't set up any appointments in advance but spent the morning at Harvard Medical School, wandering around the corridors, going into classrooms, sitting in on lectures. That same afternoon, I travelled out to Soldiers Field where Harvard Business School was located and proceeded to do the same thing, soaking up the atmosphere; I decided then and there that I would rather go into business than medicine. Being at an age where you have to justify what you do in life, I dreamed up an excuse for switching. I think that the army probably influenced my thinking, but my excuse was that medical men are, above all, firemen. When a fire breaks out, firemen arrive on the scene and try to put it out. A businessman, by contrast, doesn't have to wait for an emergency before acting. If he grows his people quickly and handles them right, he can make sure they don't get sick in the first place. That was my idealistic reason for switching from medicine to business.

I had the summer off in 1947. I had finished at McGill and knew I was heading to Harvard in the fall, and, since I hadn't managed to get there during the war, I saw it as a great opportunity to visit Europe. I had actually got as far as Halifax twice when I was in the army en route to the European theatre, only to be sent back. So, it was third time lucky when I headed to Halifax once again and boarded the Aquitania, which had switched from its wartime role as a troop carrier. I was accompanied on that voyage by plenty of other young people anxious to experience Europe just after the War.

Happenstance, once again, turned up unexpectedly when I arrived in London. I was walking down Bond Street or some other thoroughfare and who should I run into but Mr Killam, who was in London on one of his frequent business trips. He asked me what I was up to, and, without skipping a beat, he made this unusual proposal: "Do you want to go to Paris tonight?" He then reached into his pocket and pulled out two airline tickets. "Dorothy wants to go to Paris because there's a big party at the British Embassy tonight, and she doesn't want to miss it. I don't want to go, so why don't you take Dorothy?" There I was, 22 years old and just invited to a luxurious evening in Paris. I gladly took the tickets, met up with Mrs Killam, and off we flew in great style. We arrived at the legendary Georges V Hotel, just off the Champs-Elysées, where she had a huge suite, practically a whole floor. It was the way Dorothy travelled. But there was a slight problem. I hadn't set out on my summer holiday in Europe with a tuxedo. No worries, Mrs Killam assured me, "The hotel will supply you with a black tie." Sure enough, they did, but they weren't in the business of providing proper footwear. I only had one pair of shoes with me, black brogues that I had worn when I was in the Black Watch reserves back in Montreal. So off I went to the embassy ball wearing the black tie and my Black Watch brogues.

The party was going in fine style and I was standing beside Mrs Killam when she suggested, "I want you to meet Wallis Windsor." This was a time when Edward VIII's abdication and subsequent marriage to Wallis Simpson was still the stuff of scandal. To this day, I can still remember meeting her. She was one of two or three women to whom I have been introduced in my lifetime who had the ability to suddenly treat you as if there is no one else but you in the world. Some men call it being devoured, but I don't call it that. I'd call it a way of focusing. She had these penetrating blue eyes, and she really homed in on me. I asked her to dance, and while we were dancing Sir Duff Cooper, the British ambassador, turned to Mrs Killam and exclaimed, "Extraordinary shoes that young man is wearing!"

Anyway, that was I.W. Killam for you. Meets you on the street and instantly figures out a way to avoid going to Paris. He clearly didn't like parties.

Dorothy, on the other hand, who was fourteen years her husband's junior, lived for parties and saw it as her role to help spend her husband's millions. Hers was the life of the rich and famous, a social whirlwind that took her between Paris, London, New York, the French Riviera, and the Bahamas with a retinue of servants and trunks full of clothes. Later in life, after the death of her husband, Mrs Killam ended up buying the legendary La Leopolda, an over-the-top villa at Villefranche-sur-Mer overlooking Cap Ferrat on the French Riviera. Originally built by King Leopold II of Belgium for his favourite mistress, La Leopolda was later the home of Giovanni Agnelli, head of Fiat, the Italian automaker, before being sold to Mrs Killam.

The Windsors were great friends of the Killams because of their mutual association with the Bahamas. After the abdication in 1936, the duke and duchess attracted considerable criticism in Britain because of their none-too-secret Nazi sympathies, which became a source of embarrassment and more with the onset of war. Anxious to get the troublesome duke as far away from Europe as possible, Churchill shipped him off to the Bahamas as governor of the colony in 1940.

The Killams actually owned two homes in the Bahamas, one in Nassau and the other on Paradise Island, then known by the much less romantic name of Hog Island. The Nassau mansion was next door to the governor's residence, so Mrs Killam and the duchess, both American ladies of style who had married up in the world, became great pals. I first visited the Killams in the Bahamas at Christmas of 1945, just after the end of the war when I had gone back to complete my degree at McGill. I was just 21.

Christmas with the Killams in Nassau was about as far removed from the officers' training school in Brockville as one could expect. It was black tie every night, with an orchestra playing in the garden if you wanted to dance. Of course, Mr Killam wasn't there. It wasn't his thing. The day I arrived, Dorothy announced that bridge was on the calendar. "We're going to play bridge tonight and we play for quite a lot of money, so I'll stake you," she declared to me. "I don't know how much you know about bridge, but remember two things. If your partner opens and the next person passes, always say something. And secondly, never open without an ace. Unless you have at least one ace in your hand, don't make a bid." I've never played much bridge in my life, but I've always remembered those two rules.

Dorothy was a pretty good card player, but she did have a bit of an edge that the average bridge player wouldn't exactly have had easy access to. She would invite Charles Goren, the world's foremost bridge guru, to stay with her for weeks at a time. My mother told me once about playing at the table with Mrs Killam when Goren was in the room. At a tense point in the bidding, Mrs Killam called Goren over for advice on her hand, and my mother, who was playing against her, thought that that wasn't quite playing fair. Not one to let something like this pass without comment, my mother glared at Goren, who then said to Mrs Killam, "You have one swell pass."

Days with Mrs Killam on that trip passed at a particular pace, dominated as they were by long sessions with her naval architect. He had been brought down to the Bahamas with the remit to design a boat that Dorothy could use to cross over to Paradise Island where her second home was located. The stretch of water to cover was maybe 200 yards. Her instructions to the naval architect were that the boat must be capable of leaving Nassau after the governor's boat set off but still be able to arrive at Paradise Island before the governor's boat did. What she wanted was a fast launch with a lot of comfort built into it. This is how the very rich think. You should have seen the look on the architect's face as Mrs Killam kept adding weight to the boat by insisting on various comforts and luxuries. And, of course, as she added weight, it became harder and harder for him to guarantee that her launch could accelerate fast enough to beat the Windsors' to the dock.

Though the trip to the Bahamas was a lovely break, I realized that it was a bit of an unreal world, and I would have to work for a living. My MBA studies were to be financed with the help of the Canadian government through the Canadian equivalent of the GI bill, for which I am still grateful. Harvard was different from McGill but not hard to figure out. You had to work hard, which I have to admit wasn't something I had much practice doing. I never was a brilliant student. I wasn't lazy, in that I was always running or playing sports, but when it came to my studies I was not exactly committed. At Harvard, however, I shaped up and did quite well, graduating with distinction. Yet, I was never the kind of student to pull all-nighters. I'm not a night person, so I would get up at five in the morning and do my work from 5 a.m. to 7:30 a.m. I always had better ideas in the morning than I did at night.

The main emphasis in the first year at Harvard was how to work with people, to get things done through people. The first-year courses were fixed for everybody, and it was only in the second year that there were options like finance and marketing. First-year classes were divided into groups of one hundred students. The classes were nondirective and based on the case method. You would get three or four cases a night to read, and some of them were very long and complex. If you asked a professor what he thought, he would turn it right back at you. The professors weren't supposed to give their opinions but encouraged you to provide your views. After one year, frankly, we were tired of hearing our one hundred classmates talk.

In the second year, of the 625 students in the class, 400 opted for a course called Manufacturing, which was a full-year course. It was given by an extraordinary Frenchman named General Georges Doriot, a naturalized American who revolutionized the US Army's approach to research and development during the Second World War and later became known as the father of modern venture capitalism. I learned a lot from him. The general spoke English with a thick French accent, and at that first class in a big auditorium he stood up and declared, "Look, when you and I are in the same room, I talk." There was an audible sigh of relief in the room. After our first year of nondirective instruction, everybody was delighted that the professor was going to talk, and we could sit back and take notes.

After ordaining that he was the only one who would talk, Doriot continued, "We will start this class with the definition of an organization. The definition of an organization is a whole bunch of people helping one man do a job." A pretty stark way of defining things. As a result, he went on, it's good advice for those people who are working for that one man (this was 1947 after all) to have reasonable short-term goals. But, that one person also needs to have long-term goals, particularly if he is running a large company. The trick, Doriot argued, was to get those other people to think that those goals were their own. It's not standing up and saying, "We are going to do this. We are going to be number one in the world." The trick is to say, "We want to end up roughly here, and it's up to you guys to figure out how we're going to do it." It was a lesson I took to heart. What was always fun when running a big company was to see an idea that you had seeded two months earlier start coming back at you. So, as I always say, leading is an exercise in selflessness, not selfishness. The same as marriage.

Other famous lines from the general:

A real courageous man is a man who does something courageous when no one is watching him.

An auditor is like a tailor. He can make a fat man look thinner
or taller or younger.

You will get nowhere if you do not inspire people.

Always remember that someone somewhere is making a
product that will make your product obsolete.

Doriot divided his class into groups of five and gave each group
the assignment to discover a new product and tell him how one
could make a business out of that product. Doriot would then har-
vest the best ideas from the class and take them down to his own
company, American Research and Development Corp., and his
company would capitalize on those ideas. Remember Toni, the
hair care product that women used for home permanents? That
idea was from our class. Doriot ended up doing quite well with
four or five of those student concepts, but the activities of American
Research went well beyond that. The company was founded in
1946, and over the following twenty-five years it helped develop
more than one hundred start-ups, including such firms as
Digital Equipment Corp., which was started in 1957 by two MIT
engineers with a nest egg of $70,000 from Doriot's company.
When American Research liquidated its Digital stake in 1972, the
company was worth more than $400 million.

At the end of the academic year, the general would tell the class,
"I have to set an exam for you. The university demands it. So you
will write my exam on the 4th of June. The rules say that you have
to write the exam so I'm going to give you an exam. But I have to
be honest with you. I am not going to read any of your test papers.
The reason is because I have already given you your mark. The
university will tell you what your mark is after the exam. And

when you read your mark, I want you to know what it means. The mark that I give you is my guess as to whether you will succeed in business or not."

After finishing that year at Harvard, I spent the summer of 1948 at the Canadian Pulp and Paper Association's headquarters in the Sun Life Building in Montreal. It was my first real job in the business world and an eye-opener. The assignment was quite simple. Once a week I contacted all the producers that belonged to the association, blue bloods of Canadian industry like Abitibi and Bowater. It was the era when Canada was the king of newsprint producers. I would find out what products the companies had shipped the week before and at what price. I would combine these figures into some big number that no producer could use to figure out what the others were up to, and that figure was published. Over that summer I began to wonder what constituted competition in the industry. Among other things, I discovered that it was customary for competitive pulp and paper companies to have regular meetings of their foremen at which they would discuss production problems. There didn't seem to me to be much of a competitive environment at all. When I asked how the paper companies competed with each other, the only answer I could get was that it was all a question of volume. They were in a race to produce more than the other guy, which was a formula for failure because you would always end up with excess capacity. Several months later, in the winter months that followed that first year, I was offered a job in the pulp and paper industry, and I declined as politely as possible. I didn't want to work in an industry where the only thing you could do to be better than the other guy was to produce more. So I ended up in aluminum where I had plenty of competition – more than enough.

In the end, I did all right in Doriot's course and in the rest of the MBA program. I graduated with Distinction from Harvard Business School in June of 1949, which was the first time I ever got a high mark in anything. There were 625 people in that class, and of that total, no fewer than 105 requested to be interviewed by a Canadian company known as Alcan Aluminium. I still remember the dumbfounded look on the face of Duncan Campbell, who was to become a longtime friend and colleague at Alcan, when he walked into a room at Harvard and saw 105 people waiting to be interviewed. Of that crowd, thirteen joined Alcan on 1 July 1949. I was one of the lucky thirteen.

You have to go back to 1949 and a story in *Life*, the hugely popular picture magazine, to understand what a big deal Alcan was at the time. The *Life* cover article featured the construction of Alcan's huge Kitimat power and smelter development in British Columbia, an endeavour that captured the optimism and belief in progress that was strong at the time. The project was daring in its scope and daunting in its engineering. It involved turning a river around and sending it in the opposite direction to the Pacific Ocean instead of allowing it to drain inland as nature had designed it. The powerful river was rerouted and sent coursing through a ten-mile tunnel in the mountains and down half a mile to an underground power station. The Kitimat project was also a product of the Cold War, with the US government insisting that the power plant be built deep in the mountains to protect that strategic source of aluminum from the prospect of Soviet bombing. To young men in those days, Kitimat was exciting. Today, you could be shot for turning a river in a different direction, but in those days it got your heart racing.

Alcan was, for another reason, an exciting company for a young business school graduate. The company had gone into the war with, basically, the same men who had started the company in 1928. Alcan had made no money before the war, and, though a few new people had come on board since the early years, many had also been lost to the war. So the same elderly crew was still running Alcan in 1945 even though the company, due primarily to its huge expansion in Quebec, was ten times bigger than it had been in 1939. Not only was it a company engaged in a dynamic project, it was also a company with a lot of scope for young men to find good jobs and get ahead.

Alcan's culture at the time was unusual, in large part reflecting the way the company had been carved out of the Aluminum

Company of America (Alcoa) in 1928. The man still running Alcan in 1947 was Edward K. Davis, the younger brother of Arthur Vining Davis, the legendary founder of Alcoa. An abbreviated version of Arthur Vining Davis's name was bestowed on the new Saguenay River town of Arvida where much of Alcan's wartime boom took place. Arthur and Edward's father was a Congregational minister from Massachusetts, and the two boys were raised in a strict household where material possessions were rare.

In 1928, Arthur gave his brother the job of taking a variety of aluminum assets that Alcoa held outside the United States and told him to run them his own way. While Arthur rebelled against his modest roots and became a promoter supreme, Edward remained a spiritualist and a profound thinker, an unusual combination in business. In fact, Edward never liked the way his brother Arthur ran his US assets and set Alcan on a different path.

Edward K. Davis was a very private, lonely man who ran Alcan from a three-man office in Boston. He never came to Canada, where the company's operations were centred, preferring to communicate with the headquarters in Montreal by mail. In fact, Mr Davis would have "out-Killamed" Killam with regard to being a private person. Yet Mr Davis was one of the world's original thinkers on business organization. Some of Edward Davis's writings in the late 1940s on how business should be organized are classics.

While Mr Davis remained back in Boston, he sent an American named R. E. (Rip) Powell to Canada to run the day-to-day operations as president of Aluminum Co. of Canada. And, it was Rip Powell who became the real builder of Alcan in Canada. Powell, who hailed from Table Grove, Illinois, attended Monmouth College but never graduated and instead began working for Alcoa selling aluminum pots and pans. As a pioneer of the modern aluminum industry, Arthur Davis had found that, even though aluminum was recognized as a miracle metal, people weren't interested in buying a metal. But, they were interested in buying something like an aluminum kettle, a welcome innovation because of its ability to transmit heat quickly. So Alcoa got into the aluminum kitchenware business.

The aluminum kettle story was repeated many times subsequently. You always had to find new uses for aluminum and develop a product that would be better than one made with other materials. It was the same story with beer cans, aluminum siding, and automotive parts. You had to do everything the first time, take an aluminum ingot and fashion it into a useful end product. Then when others got into the business for these new products, you'd back out of the market. Alcan was still doing the same thing in my day. At one point in my career we were the biggest builders of private homes in Canada. Alcan Design Homes was building 6,000 houses a year. We were only doing it to demonstrate to established homebuilders that if they used aluminum windows, doors, and siding in their houses they would sell as fast as Alcan homes were. And, as soon as the use of aluminum went mainstream in homebuilding, we got out of the business.

As for Rip Powell, he got his start selling pots and pans door to door in the US Midwest. He would take a train, get off at the first stop, sell his wares, get back on the train, get off at the next stop, sell some more pots and pans, and so on. He soon proved himself to be much more than a motivated salesman but a consummate businessman as well.

Rip Powell was not just the boss of Alcan in Canada. He also became my father-in-law in September of 1949 when I married his daughter Mary. It turns out that Mary and I had the same piano teacher when I was five or six years old or so, and that's where the connection was first made. Mary arrived in Montreal as a little girl with her family in 1929 and went to Roslyn School and then to Miss Edgar's & Miss Cramp's, a girls' school in Westmount, before attending McGill. Mary spent the war years working at the National Research Council. We first met in 1939 or 1940 skiing at Mont Tremblant, but we didn't start going out seriously until well after the war, in 1948. We got married in Montreal in September of 1949. I was twenty-four and Mary was twenty-three.

But my decision to join Alcan when I finished Harvard had little to do with my future bride or her father. I decided for the same reason the other twelve guys did. I used to say that I've got a bit of an advantage because I'm married to the boss's daughter. We used to laugh about this, but what people might have said about my choice of spouse never bothered me.

It was Mr Powell (and that's what I always called him) who drove the huge expansion of the company that fed the insatiable appetite for aluminum in Britain and the US resulting from the war effort and the need to build combat aircraft. It was an effort that even today takes the breath away. Alcan built the massive Shipshaw hydroelectric dam in the Saguenay region in something like eighteen months in 1942–43 with 43,000 men on the job. Forced by circumstances to innovate, Alcan engineers developed a unique way of blocking the river flowing out of Lac Saint-Jean. The lake was a huge natural water reservoir and the overflow poured in huge volumes into the Saguenay River through a very narrow slot. What Alcan did was build a massive concrete profile of the riverbed that was stood on its end on the riverbank, and then dropped into place with explosives, instantly blocking the flow.

Alcan was back doing similarly heroic things with its Kitimat project not long after the end of the war, when I was hired. The company brought us all on as trainee managers. In those days, trainees were sent to different plants to learn how each facility worked. I started that process in the summer of 1949 and was sent to Arvida and to our plant in Etobicoke, in suburban Toronto, but sometime in August or early September I got a call and was told I would be off to the Centre d'Études Industrielles, a remarkable business school in Geneva that Edward K. Davis had founded just three years earlier.

Unhappy with Alcan's conventional trainee program, Davis saw the school as a way of speeding up the indoctrination process for new managers. After all, we were ten times the size that we used to be but still had the same managers. And again, only an American would have thought of this. Because of the company's far-flung operations, Davis believed Alcan managers should have an international understanding of business, so he preferred to base the school in Europe rather than North America. And, because many of Alcan's key assets were located in the French-speaking part of

Canada, he thought the institute should be in a French-speaking city. Geneva filled the bill.

The man Edward Davis chose to run his new institute was Paul Haenni, a Swiss research scientist who was running Alcan's research lab in Kingston, Ontario. Davis had been dreaming of building the next Arvida and decided it should be in China, at the site on the Yangtze River that would eventually become the Three Gorges power project. In pursuit of that dream, Alcan hired thirty Chinese engineers and brought them to North America in 1946 to train them in the aluminum business and get them ready to build a great Chinese aluminum smelter. The engineers were sent to Kingston to be trained under Dr Haenni.

As part of the assignment, the visiting engineers were required to write a letter every Friday to a man named Edwin J. Mejia, who had been appointed by Davis to run Alcan's Personnel Department, another corporate innovation at the time. It turned out that every Thursday night Dr Haenni invited the Chinese visitors to his home in Kingston for dinner where they discussed not just aluminum but philosophy, politics, economics, art, and the evolution of human thought. The next day they would all recount to Mr Mejia in New York how much they had learned from their host. When Edward Davis asked Mejia to find him a good man to run Alcan's new institute in Geneva, he had all these letters from the Chinese engineers telling him what they had learned from Dr Haenni. As a result of the kudos, Dr Haenni got the job of starting the school, and the first crop of students came on in 1947. Mr Davis never got to visit the school. He died that same year.

Two years later, in September of 1949, I joined as part of a fresh intake of fifteen students. For Mary and me, it meant a bit of a rush to the altar. Our planned wedding date of 1 October had to be pushed forward to 20 September. After getting married at St James the Apostle Anglican Church in downtown Montreal and celebrating at a reception at the Powell home on Doctor Penfield Avenue, we hopped on a train that night for New York and a ship the following day to Europe.

In its calendar of courses, a slim volume of less than forty pages, the Centre laid out its raison d'être in what we today would call a mission statement that began with the following words: "The *Centre d'Études Industrielles* is a post-graduate school where the functions of modern international industry are examined and studied with the object of accelerating the development of persons aspiring to assume managerial positions in this field. These studies, supplemented by field trips and special lectures, are calculated to enhance the student's ability to succeed in managerial positions."

Writing home to my mother in November of 1949, this is how I described the school: "You ask about the school and what we are studying. The aim has nothing to do with aluminum, but rather to produce a course of study focused on the international aspects of international business administration. To do this, they endeavour to make us internationally minded. This is difficult. 'Scratch the surface of an internationalist and you uncover a provincialist.' So we are situated here in Geneva because it is truly an international city. We have field training in the summer that takes us around to many different countries. We have a large number of special lectures, and make a field trip once every two weeks. Next Wednesday we go to the north of Switzerland to the Longines watch factory. The school is young. I believe that each year improvements are made. We have an excellent group of students, and much of the success of the work depends on them."

Courses were given on industrial finance, international monetary policy, international labour legislation, and other "big" issues, but there was also a fascinating roster of guest lecturers. Visiting speakers were a big part of what the school did, and I think they should be part of every business school. The first visiting lecturer that Dr Haenni brought to the school turned out to be a distant relative of his, a defrocked Catholic priest who had been excommunicated because of his Communist sympathies. It was Dr Haenni's way of letting us know we were going to have to meet all kinds of people in the world. It was hardly the kind of guest you'd meet at Harvard Business School. The topics were always challenging. A Prof. Rappard spoke to us on "the movement for a European Union" when it was still in its most embryonic stage, and a Prof. Golay lectured on the "psychology of cartels."

The program was also innovative in that it included a series of industrial visits, including several to textile plants and steel mills. I remember going down a coal mine in France and being surrounded by Polish miners who were naked except for their helmets and searchlights. The heat was awful. We were down on the ground, crawling on our bellies through tiny tunnels. Talk about claustrophobic! Then in the summer of 1950, I spent a lot of time in England visiting Alcan's plants there. I came away from that experience with a lifelong distaste for what I call "the white coats," the very British practice of differentiating employees by classification. A British plant with maybe 800 workers might have three or four different dining rooms with the one you ate in dependent on where you were slotted into the management structure. There was too much formality. You could only speak to people in your own particular field. I found this class system oppressive, but it seemed to be accepted by everybody else in the British facilities.

Although I was a fulltime student while in Geneva, I was still on Alcan's payroll and being paid the princely sum of 425 Swiss francs a month. But the only decent apartment my new wife and I could find cost 400 Swiss francs a month, so the first year we didn't manage to balance the family budget. It was nevertheless a pretty romantic way to start our marriage. Our flat was a fifth-floor walkup in Geneva's Vieille Ville that we rented from the owner of an antique shop. It was located at "the top of a hill in the distinguished part of Geneva," as I described in a letter to my parents. "There is no elevator – just winding stairs and so the climb is great – a fact which helps to explain why we were able to get it. Thus it deserves the name penthouse." I readily admitted that the flat was "too expensive for us. But after seeing some of the grim places being offered, we were able to rationalize ourselves into it by spending some of our leftover honeymoon money on it. I hope you agree that the decision was okay. With the high cost of living in Geneva (about twice Montreal for everything) we do not expect to save."

We may have come from different countries and backgrounds but all of us were embarking on our careers and married lives together. Among the fifteen students that year, we produced nine babies. Only one of the students had a car, and it was his job to drive all of the expectant mothers to the clinic to give birth. Every time he did so, he would paint another baby on the hood of his car. When it was time for Mary and me to make that trip to the clinic, I found out that it was against Swiss law to keep the husband out of the delivery room.

We arrived at the clinic around midnight. The doctor arrived about thirty minutes later, examined Mary, and turned to me and said, "I think you and I are going to go for a walk." He took me out into the streets of Geneva and we walked for two solid hours, getting further and further away from the clinic. I was getting more and more fussed about this and asked, "Why are we doing this?" And he said, "It's not going to be an easy birth and if we hang around we run the risk of doing something we shouldn't do, so we're taking a long walk to make sure we don't do anything we shouldn't do." We got back around four in the morning. Then he picked up a canister and a mask and turned a few dials, put the mask over his own face and inhaled deeply. I was astonished and beginning to think he was putting himself under, but then he gave me a little wink and said, "It doesn't do much."

Anyway, I felt that for the next two hours I was on the one-yard line of Harvard defending against Yale, but everything went well, and, after a night of hard work for Mary, our first child was born on 4 January 1951. Michael weighed ten pounds, six ounces. We soon found out that he was ineligible to be a Swiss citizen. A child's grandfather has to be Swiss for the child to be considered a Swiss citizen, and it doesn't matter if the baby is born there. One of the reasons I eventually wanted to leave Geneva is that you're always considered an outsider in Switzerland.

The Swiss gave special meaning to the expression uptight. Geneva was full of signs saying, "Keep off the grass," or "Don't park here." Don't do this and don't do that. We used to joke that Geneva's civic motto was "Ce qui n'est pas défendu est interdit."

But the Genevois were very accommodating and polite. Though they were welcoming, they never gave you a feeling of really belonging there politically or socially. After three years in Geneva, Mary once described Switzerland as a chocolate box full of potatoes.

One day when I was working at the school, Mary drove by to pick me up after work. She recounted to me how on the way to school, on a narrow street with stone walls on both sides, a kid on a bicycle had suddenly darted out of a side street and hit our car. The collision didn't damage the car much, but it bent one wheel of the kid's bicycle out of shape. Before she could get out of the car and see how he was doing, he had disappeared. I said to myself, "If I know the Swiss, we'd better stop at the police station on the way home and report it." At the main police station, I reported that my wife had been run into by a kid on a bicycle who got up, took his damaged bike, and disappeared. Sure enough, in the newspaper the next day there was a story about an "étrangère" who had collided with a bicycle and left the scene of the accident.

I called the Swiss Touring Club and sought out their opinion. They volunteered that the President of the Club was a lawyer and would take care of it. That didn't stop Mary from being charged with hit and run. When her day in court arrived, the first thing I did was produce the officer from the local police station to whom we had first reported the incident, and he duly testified that I had come in and given an account of what happened. In the end, Mary was fined sixty francs.

But, what was really funny was the case that came just before ours. A local man had been driving home in the rain on the outskirts of Geneva, and his car had skidded off the slippery road and gone into a ditch. A policeman on his bicycle came by, stopped, and charged the man with reckless driving. He had the same lawyer as we did, who told him to let him do the talking in court and not say anything. His client wouldn't listen. He stood up and berated the policeman, saying that instead of thinking about how to help get the car back on the road, all the policeman had been thinking about was what crime to charge him with. He went on and on bawling out the policeman. The judge eventually fined him ten francs. Then the man embarked on another diatribe about how absolutely ridiculous the ten-franc fine was. After about five minutes, the man said he would be willing to pay five francs but ten was "ridiculous." The judge responded, "Five francs it is. Case closed." If we had been more belligerent, maybe Mary would have got off with a smaller fine.

The course lasted only a year, but as the program was ending I was told that I would be staying on at the Centre as a member of the staff. It wasn't my choice. I figured I had had enough of school and university, including my stint at officer training school in the army, and wanted to go to work in a real job. Instead, I was assigned to help administer the Centre, organize field trips, and teach one course on administrative practices based on the Harvard Business School's case method. In assessing my personality at the end of the program, the administrators included my main characteristics as being: "intelligent, imaginative. Conscientious, sociable, human, fine personality, solid education, organized mind, good psychologist, retiring, somewhat stiff, not very aggressive." It was a bit over-the-top, but of all the words of flattery, the one that meant the most to me was that simple word, "human."

I could have stayed on in Geneva, but I felt that it was important to broaden my experience. In the spring of my second year on staff at the Centre, I told Dr Haenni that it was time for me to do some ordinary commercial work at Alcan. He told me that the president of Alcan's sales company in New York, Ward Van Alstyne, was coming through Geneva in a couple of weeks and suggested that I ask him for a job. I made my pitch to Van Alstyne, and, to my horror, he told me that he was looking for somebody to work in the company's advertising department. The problem was that I knew who the advertising manager was. He was a nice guy but definitely not exciting, and I knew that advertising was the least important part of an aluminum ingot sales company in New York. We were not dependent on advertising and spent little or no money on it. But, I had one of those ten-second moments in life when I knew that if I said no, I would probably never go very far in Alcan.

I'd have stayed on at the school in Geneva indefinitely. So I responded quickly and enthusiastically, "I'd like to do that, Mr Van Alstyne."

I often use that vignette as an example for young people embarking on their careers. When you're offered your first job, pay no attention to what it is. Instead, ask yourself, "Is it the right company? Is the right person running that company?" If you can say yes to both, then ignore the actual job description and take the plunge. It turns out that New York was the perfect place for me to start. In June of 1952, I arrived at the Alcan sales office and Van Alstyne told me that they had changed their minds about my work in advertising and were going to give me a sales territory, which was perfect. That's how I got started.

3

"We Were Like the Jesuits"

Selling Aluminum to the World

With my adventure in Geneva over, it was time to start a real career. It was nice for both Mary and me to be closer to family in Montreal, but we knew that life in New York City with a young family was going to be a challenge. We had one small child, Michael, who had been born in Geneva, and another one was due in a few months. A cramped apartment in Manhattan simply didn't seem like an attractive option, so we decided to live well outside of the city in an area that was good for raising kids. We ended up in Peapack, New Jersey, a pristine village in the bucolic Somerset Hills seventy kilometres from Manhattan, where we rented an eighteenth century house on an owner-operated farm. It was in the centre of New Jersey's horse country and popular with New Yorkers anxious to escape the city on weekends. Jacqueline Kennedy Onassis later had a weekend home in Peapack, which she initially rented in 1965 and later purchased. It was only sold by the Kennedy family after her death in 1994. We ended up living in Peapack for four years. It was a great place for a young family. I can still remember the night I came home to tell Mary that we were moving back to Montreal and she burst into tears. She didn't want to leave.

Yet, despite the pleasures of life in the country, my daily commute into New York was quite the ordeal. On a good day it would take two hours and five minutes door to door each way. I had a $450, thirdhand Chevy that I would take to the train station. From there, I took a fifty-five-minute train ride to Hoboken on the Delaware, Lackawanna & Western Railroad, the D L & W, which we commuters referred to, from unfortunate experience, as the "Delay, Linger and Wait." Then there was an awful twenty-minute subway ride under the Hudson River into Manhattan, where I often thought that my life would end in a deadly crash as that infernal train hurtled through a darkened tunnel. After emerging from that hellhole, my commute was capped by a final twenty-minute ride up to Rockefeller Center on the I R T subway line. There was no air conditioning on the subway, so on a hot day I would arrive at the office feeling like a sodden rag. If I didn't leave by 5:15 p.m., I had to spend the night in New York. When a late afternoon business meeting left me with no choice, I would check into the Harvard Club where they charged $1.00 a night for a bed. During the war, the Club had boarded over its indoor swimming pool and turned it into a makeshift dormitory filled with cots so that they could accommodate guys like me who got stranded in New York. That dormitory was still in place a decade later.

As for the work, it was an eye-opener. My job was to sell rail carload lots of aluminum ingot and aluminum extrusion billets. Most of my clients were individual fabricators in the northeast US, independent manufacturers who could buy one extrusion press and be in business making windows, doors and even rabbit-ear antennae for T V sets a few weeks later after a capital expenditure of less than a million dollars. The great thing about the extrusion process is that it's a very cheap and quick way to get a metal shape. You have to spend a lot of money to customize the mould, but once you have it you just squirt the aluminum out like toothpaste. For these independents, who owned hard assets of less than a million dollars, the minimum carload of aluminum ingot might cost $50,000, a major amount of money, so credit was a big problem.

Alcan's competitors in the business were the three big US aluminum producers, Alcoa, Reynolds, and Kaiser. But, Alcan was in a unique position; unlike the other three, who all made aluminum extrusions in competition with the independents, Alcan was a primary producer only, which built loyalty with these customers.

Whenever there was a surplus of aluminum, Alcoa, Reynolds, and Kaiser would go to the US government and ask it to protect the industry and not let Canadian-made ingot into the US. They would become extremely protectionist. Our reaction was to go to all the independents and urge them to call their congressmen and senators and tell them that if they excluded Canadian ingot, they would be shutting out the only supplier who wasn't competing directly with them.

Because many of these independents were small businesses, they were often the most credit risky of customers. I remember the first time that I went to a customer who owed us money. It was down near Philadelphia, in an area I had never visited before. I drove my car up to this little plant, and there were two spanking new Cadillacs parked outside. I went in to see the customer and told him that I was there to collect the bill. He got red in the face, told me to tell my boss where to get off and then spat out that they didn't always have the cash on hand to pay us. Not convinced of my customer's poverty, I ventured, "How about the two Cadillacs parked out there?" The customer was clearly not pleased. "Now listen, sonny, grow up, those cars are in the wife's name." So I grew up to learn quickly what, for certain businessmen, ends up in the wife's name.

New York also proved a useful training ground in the art of handling alcohol at work. This being the fifties, social drinking was an essential element of business relationships. Although I didn't drink much in those days and was never much interested in the three-martini lunch, I must admit I was never opposed to having one martini. On my first day on the job in 1952, my boss asked me to take one of Alcan's rough and tough customers to lunch. Having been either in school or the army all my life to that point, I was a bit of a babe in the woods when it came to drinking during the workday. My boss said, "Look, I don't want to tell you how to behave, but this guy is going to want three martinis at lunch. My advice to you is when he orders a martini, you order a gin on the rocks." I was perplexed and asked my boss what possible difference this could make. He responded, "They'll put two and a half ounces of gin in each of his martinis. But if you order a gin on the rocks, you'll get an ounce and a quarter of gin and a lot of ice. He'll think you're a real drinker, and you can just sip that one drink all through the meal as the ice melts." That's exactly how the lunch went. I took the client to a restaurant on Madison Avenue in the advertising district and as he went through his three martinis, I slowly worked on my ounce and a quarter of gin. We were sitting in a booth that had high sides, and in the next booth I could hear two advertising guys talking, but I couldn't see them. They were having a very heated discussion about whether or not to hire some guy named Jack. One of them was for it and the other was against. Their discussion went on and on, and finally came a phrase that I've never forgotten. One of them said, "Okay, I'll admit that Jack is smart. But tell me, how does he stack up wisdom-wise?" Madison Avenue language, I admit. How does he stack up wisdom-wise? But to the point. It's a phrase I've used countless times in my life since.

The Alcan culture did not exactly encourage excessive alcohol consumption. The father of Arthur and Edward Davis had been a Congregational Church minister in Massachusetts, and that abstemious tradition continued at Alcan where Nathanael Davis, Edward's son, was very much against having any alcohol in the office. When Alcan moved into Place Ville Marie in 1963, we had a very nice executive dining room. Nat tried valiantly to keep it alcohol free, but we would often have business guests for lunch and they would want a drink. Nat gave in and made Campari, but only Campari, available. That lasted until a marvellous outside director, Bill Twaits, the C E O of Imperial Oil, stood up at one of the board meetings and made a great speech about why the directors should be able to have a martini at lunch in the dining room. One of the most effective presentations I've ever heard from an outside director anywhere! And for once, senior management listened.

After four years in the US, during which we expanded our family to three children, (the fourth was born a year after we got back to Canada) it was time to head home to Montreal. In September of

1956 I was offered the number two job in worldwide sales. One of Edward Davis' unusual inventions was a staff sales organization as well as a line sales organization. It was kind of complex. In fact, I later spent a lot of my career going back to a much simpler organization than the one I inherited when I started. I moved back to Montreal to an office in the Sun Life Building, reporting to the head of sales in New York, Elmer MacDowell, who had been selling aluminum for decades, starting at Alcoa.

Despite the occasional late payment problem, we had few bad debts in the US. In the booming fifties, a lot of these independents grew very fast, and as they grew they bought more and more aluminum from us. When I started as a salesman in 1952, aluminum was in short supply so I was calling on customers but couldn't offer them what they wanted to buy. Then in 1957, the market turned sharply in the other direction, and we had more metal than we could sell. It's then that the years of relationship building paid off. A lot of our customers recalled that we had been there for them even when supply conditions were really tight. They would tell us, "You came around and helped us even though you couldn't sell us much of anything, so now we'll buy from you."

There I was at thirty-two, suddenly in charge of a couple of hundred sales people around the world. It was a big jump for me and a generational shock for my employees because John Bueb, the man I was replacing, was in his sixties and off to retirement. But my immediate challenge was to deal with Ronald Kinsman, a colourful character at Alcan who had expected to get the job.

I remember my first day in Montreal in what had been Mr Bueb's office, a much bigger office than I'd ever had, and in walks Ronald Kinsman. He was an amateur actor, and, with many people like that, an encounter of any kind at any time is the perfect excuse for a stage entrance. He appeared in my office in dramatic fashion with, as always, a handkerchief hanging out of his cuff, and the first thing he said to me was, "Mr Culver, do you think it is appropriate for your vice president to be spending his evenings lounging on a sofa at the top of Mount Royal with the wife of your chief accountant?" I figured that he must have been acting in some play with the Montreal Repertory Theatre, which had its play-house on the mountain, so, with my rapier wit, I responded, "Well, Mr Kinsman, it takes all kinds of people to run a business."

In the end, Kinsman stayed on and was a great help and support. I will be forever grateful to him for solving the secretary problem. In moving into the Montreal sales job, I inherited a lovely lady for the position, but one whom I knew from the start would not work out for me. I didn't know what to do about it. Then Kinsman came into my office one day and said to me, "I think you should take Miss Bowen, who's my secretary, and I'll find someone else." It proved an excellent arrangement. Miss Bowen remained with me as my assistant from 1956 until 1983, a smart woman and the ultimate gatekeeper who instilled the kind of fear in managers that I never was able to engender. By the time Miss Bowen decided to retire and move back to her native England in 1983, she had already chosen her replacement. Janice Darrah was a capable young woman from Quebec's Eastern Townships who had been working at Alcan for Eric West, an executive vice president. After a period of training under Miss Bowen, Janice became my trusted assistant, first at Alcan and then at my investment firm. So from 1956 to 2013, a total of fifty-seven years, I have had only two assistants, and the second one was chosen by the first. My good fortune knows no bounds.

I had suddenly become a boss and had the job of figuring out how to sell aluminum around the world. I've always been a great believer in doing walkabouts as a basic element of good management, but in the 1950s international air travel was still in its infancy, so a walkabout through a global sales organization like Alcan's was going to be a challenge. A trip to Europe took two weeks, for example. There was none of this flying out on a Sunday night from North America and returning on Friday in time for the weekend. I only once took a ship across the Atlantic, and that's a story in itself.

In the winter of 1957, I flew to Europe to spend two weeks visiting Alcan's sales operation and decided that since I'd have a lot of reports to write at the end of the trip I'd sail on the Queen

Elizabeth on the way back. After the ship docked in New York, I would report on my European foray to Mr MacDowell at the Alcan sales office and then head home to Montreal. It was an experiment I did once but was never to repeat. By the time I got on the Queen Elizabeth in Southampton I was worn out from my whirlwind European trip, so much so that I didn't show up in the dining room until lunchtime the next day. I was immediately asked whether I wanted to sit by myself or at a bigger table. I told the maître d' that I'd prefer to be more sociable, so I was placed at a table of about eight people next to a man who turned out to be the advertising manager for Coca-Cola Export. I remember him telling the waiter at that first lunch, "Every time you see me sitting at this table, you bring over some caviar. Every time." I figured out that the advertising manager for Coca-Cola enjoyed the better things in life.

In a dining room aboard ship there's always a certain amount of background noise, a constant hum of conversation and the clinking of dishes and glasses. During that first lunch, all of a sudden the noise stopped and there was a hush. I looked around, and the most extraordinary looking lady was walking into the dining room. A woman of a certain age. Not particularly good looking but very striking. Everyone had stopped eating and was watching her. She walked over to the captain's table and sat down. Then we all went back to our lunch again.

That evening, I was sitting at the same table and again there was a hush as she walked into the dining room. This time she was wearing a long white dress with a collar that rose above her neck in two sharp peaks, making her look like a character out of a Walt Disney movie, and, to my absolute horror, instead of heading for the captain's table she made a beeline for me! "You're Mr Culver?" she inquired. When I nodded, she asked, "Where is Mr MacDowell?" I suddenly remembered that MacDowell, my boss at Alcan, had told me that he usually took the same ship that sailed every 7 February from Southampton. This was obviously a lady with whom MacDowell had spent some time on his annual sales trips to Europe. "I see that you work for the same company as

Mr MacDowell, but where is he?" she continued. When I explained that I was replacing him this year, she asked me to stick around after dinner. "We have a group upstairs, so join us for some dancing," she said. I soon discovered that this striking woman ran a fancy dress shop next door to New York's St Regis Hotel, and the boutique was known by the wonderfully evocative name Henry à la Pensée. She went on a buying trip to Europe every year and always took the Queen Elizabeth home on its early February sailing from Southampton. In her company onboard was a coterie of dress buyers from Saks Fifth Avenue, Lord & Taylor, and other high-end stores, who travelled to Europe to see the latest fashions. They played bridge all day, and they drank champagne and danced all night.

After joining in the revelry, I soon became really exhausted! I don't think I had the time or energy to write a single word of the reports that I had planned to work on. To make things worse, about halfway across the Atlantic we were told that there was a tugboat strike in New York, which meant we couldn't dock there and would have to go to Halifax instead. The five-day trip became a seven-day trip, as the captain slowed the ship in the vain hope that the tugboat strike would end, and the parties went on and on. These ladies were the early glass ceiling types. They worked like men, and they played like men. I was exhausted by the time we docked in Halifax. I took a plane back to Montreal, and a day or so later I took the train down to New York to report to Mr MacDowell on the results of my trip. Before seeing him, I wondered whether to mention the lady from Henry à la Pensée or just forget about it. I decided to be totally natural. "Well Mr MacDowell, I had quite a trip home on the Queen E mostly due to a friend of yours who goes by the name Madame à la Pensée." His face was impassive. "Charming lady, don't you think?" And I responded, "Yes, indeed," and that was the end of that conversation. That was the only time I went by ship on a business trip, and I said that I'd never do it again. All that partying was simply too draining.

Instead, I became a frequent flyer in the days when air travel was noisy and time consuming but always something of an adventure.

That early travel was in D C -3s, D C -4s, and D C -7s, and I remember thinking that we would never, ever need a better airplane than a Lockheed Constellation. It was on one of those trans-Atlantic flights that I had an interesting encounter with C.D. Howe, the legendary "Minister of Everything" in the federal government of the 1940s and 1950s. He was responsible for much of the formidable industrial effort that accompanied Canada's military role in the Second World War. We met at London's Savoy Hotel and drove out to Heathrow airport together to catch the same flight to Montreal. During the flight, Howe told me that he and his wife, whom he always referred to as Mrs Howe, had decided that their house on the upper reaches of Mountain Street in downtown Montreal had become too large for the two of them. The Howes called their seven grown children together on a Wednesday night and announced that the house had been sold and that they were moving into an apartment. He told them that he was taking Mrs Howe away for the weekend that Friday and they would be home at 4 p.m. on the Monday. He then set out the terms of an unusual offer to his seven sons and daughters. "You can take anything out of the house you like as long as it is gone by 4 p.m. on Monday." Mr Howe continued, "When we came home on Monday, as I was putting the key in the lock I said to Mrs Howe, 'I wonder what the house is going to look like?' We opened the door, and walked in. Nothing had changed. Everything was exactly as we had left it." He then turned to his wife and said, "Well, we must admit that our children aren't very acquisitive. They haven't taken a thing. We'd better have a glass of wine to celebrate." So, he continued to me, "I went down to the wine cellar and it was empty." Not a bottle was left. The one thing the Howe siblings could divide by seven without having a fight was the wine cellar.

In early October 1957, I left Montreal on my first full walkabout trip around the world. The trek started in a D C -3 with initial stops in Toronto, Winnipeg, Calgary, and Vancouver. There I switched to a Canadian Pacific Airlines D C -4, which took eight hours to fly from Vancouver to Cold Bay, Alaska where we stopped for fuel. The D C -4 was a propeller-driven plane that belched fire and shook constantly. As in an old train, there was one pull-down berth over every four seats, and for an extra $75 you could rent the berth and have a sleep. After we left Cold Bay, I climbed up into my berth, put on my pyjamas, and slept for eight hours, after which I figured I'd broken the back of the trip. I got dressed, slipped down out of the berth, went up to the front and opened the curtain where there was a place for four people to sit, and there was a light on. The rest of the plane was in total darkness, and the navigator was sitting there alone. "Well, we must be getting close," I offered hopefully. He looked at his watch and said, "We've got another six hours and fifty-four minutes. We're now approaching the Russian coastline, and we're being followed by Russian radar. I hope we're on the right track." Total travel time between Cold Bay and Tokyo, 14 hours and 54 minutes.

After a week in Japan, I got on the famous Pan Am Flight One, which used to start in New York and fly around the world. I embarked from Tokyo at midnight, having been entertained at a pretty good dinner earlier that evening. I slipped into the aisle seat beneath the berth that I'd booked, and sitting in the dark next to me was a young Canadian woman. I started talking with her and asked her where she was going. She responded, "I'm on my way to Hong Kong to meet my new husband." I said, "What do you mean your new husband?" She explained, "I've just married a man who is working in Pakistan. He couldn't come home for the marriage so his brother stood in as proxy for him at the wedding yesterday in Toronto. I had to be married or I couldn't go to Pakistan with him. I could only get into the country legally if I was his wife." The couple hadn't seen each other in eight months and was scheduled to reunite in Hong Kong. I pointed at the berth above us and said, "You take the berth. I'm not meeting anybody in Hong Kong, and you'd better have a good sleep." So she went up and fell asleep in the berth.

The next morning arrived with brilliant sunshine. About an hour out of Hong Kong, I saw the skipper, a nice looking American pilot of about sixty years old, walking toward the washrooms at the back of the plane. When he emerged after about fifteen minutes he stopped and said to me, "I've just had a good shave and I'm ready for a long day." I said, "What's the problem?" He responded, "Bad weather in Hong Kong." The pilot explained that the only alternative was Manila, five hours of flying beyond Hong Kong. He would first attempt to land in Hong Kong, but if the weather wasn't good he'd pull up. "There are a lot of other planes in the same predicament. I'm the check pilot for landings in Hong Kong, which is what I do when I'm not flying around the world. So, if I decide not to land we'll have plenty of company going down to Manila. If I quit, they will too." We started down. The plane was bouncing around, and suddenly the air conditioning went on the blink and the temperature began rising fast. It was one of the few times I've ever had on a plane when I really wondered if we'd emerge from the ordeal. Then one of the flight attendants fainted in the aisle, and just then the lady behind me stood up and declared in a loud voice, "I'm not scared. I'm a Catholic!"

We made two attempts to land at Hong Kong airport and both times the pilot pulled up, so off we went to Manila. By the time we got back to Hong Kong twelve hours later, everybody in the plane knew the story of the young woman I'd sent up to the berth and how she was going to be met in Hong Kong by the new husband she hadn't seen for eight months. When we finally landed, we all were hanging back to see the great reunion take place. When the couple did meet up, the passengers all broke out in applause. Just like in the movies! In the end, I was away for nine weeks circling the globe and arrived home just ten days before our last child, Mark, was born.

The sales organization I took over in 1956 was, admittedly, a little sedentary. Edward Davis's structure meant that there was a series of overlapping arrangements that I found confusing. What I felt then and still believe profoundly is that it should be very clear who's in charge of what and that there should be very few layers of management. At about that time, I was at a dinner somewhere in the Maritimes and seated beside a bishop. I said to him, "As a businessman, I really admire the organization of the Catholic Church."

He asked me what I admired about it. I responded that, "I admire the fact that you're a huge organization with only four layers of management: priest, bishop, cardinal, pope." The bishop shot back, "You're wrong. There are only three layers of management in the Catholic Church: priest, bishop, pope." Then he looked at me with a smile and said, "I'll admit that whenever I go to see His Holiness with a problem, he sends me to see a cardinal."

I like the idea of few layers of management and clear geographical mandates. I used to say to the people running Alcan's geographical areas, "I don't want to hear about things that you can feel and touch and move. Don't ask me whether it would be a good idea to shut one plant or open another or a good idea to move a piece of equipment ten feet from one side to another. But anything that you can't touch or feel, I do want to hear about. Anything which is strategy, ethics, all the things that are invisible, I want to hear about, but I don't want to hear about the hardware side of it."

Arriving in that sales job at head office, my goal was to increase the top line by increasing revenue, meaning I was what I would call a "hunter." Within a year of arriving back in Montreal, for the first time since the start of the Second World War, we entered into a period when aluminum was in oversupply, and we weren't getting the revenue we were hoping for. Because of our low power cost, it didn't make sense to cut back smelting capacity unless we really had to. I always felt it was up to someone else in the business with higher costs to cut back. The trick was to find markets for the metal. Until that point we had been a producer's producer, making ingot and selling it to people who fabricated it. But with the arrival of Reynolds, Kaiser, and others in the US aluminum industry, we had to begin finding ways of going downstream in order to get secure outlets for our own aluminum. That's what occupied most of my time from 1956 to 1975, when I became president of Aluminum Company of Canada. I used to say that if you do something that other people can also do and you do it extremely well, you can make a living, but if you can also do some things that other people cannot do, you can make a good living. So, research and downstream development were the key elements of what we were working on in those days. That's when we started putting aluminum into beverage cans, into castings for automobiles, and other uses.

That created new challenges for Alcan, and by the early 1960s we had plants in many different locations in the United States. As we acquired small cable plants and engaged in various downstream activities, I started sending people all over the United States, often to facilities in hard-to-reach places. Since I didn't have an unlimited supply of talent, in 1964 I figured it was time that Alcan had an airplane to move people around and get the experts quickly to the places where they were needed. I even had a particular plane in mind, a new Hawker Siddeley 125 business jet with Viper engines, which was going to set Alcan back $734,000 for a basic aircraft, with the custom interior not included. I knew it was not going to be an easy sell to the management committee, a pretty conservative group of about fifteen managers. When the day came to make my proposal, I had all of my arguments lined up and I presented them with whatever skill I could muster, but, as I scanned the sceptical faces around the table, I soon realized that I was getting absolutely nowhere. For the management committee, an airplane was an extravagance that would set a bad example given that we were constantly lecturing our people about reducing costs. Alcan was a company that had never even owned its own head office premises let alone an airplane.

Seeing that I was not winning over the management committee, I looked around the room and there was Scotty Bruce, president of Aluminum Company of Canada. Scotty was an instinct manager, a man who managed from the gut. You might have occasionally criticized him for his methods but never for the reason behind them. He had a feel for what was the right thing to do. I can remember being in Scotty Bruce's office one day when his secretary came in and told him that Prime Minister Pearson was on the phone. I asked him whether I should leave and he said no. Scotty listened to Pearson for a while and then, to my discomfort, began berating the prime minister in quite harsh tones. "Don't ask me to raise money for the widow of Guy Favreau [the late justice minister] if you insist upon keeping the death duty in place, which is the reason she needs help in the first place. Get rid of the death duty, and I'll raise any amount of money you want for Mrs Favreau, but I won't do anything until you do it." Not long after that the federal government eliminated death duties.

Scanning the room, I decided my only chance was to appeal directly to Scotty Bruce about the airplane. Moving off my prepared remarks, I told the group, "Gentlemen, I now have to send our guys to many small towns in the US where we have manufacturing activities, and I want to make sure those men are able to be home at night in bed with their wives." At which point Scotty Bruce interrupted and said, "Culver is right. That's the reason to buy the airplane!" We took the plunge and bought it. Right from the start I made sure the plane was not to be used just by the high command but by anybody in the company who needed it for a fruitful purpose. For this to happen, I said that my office would pay for the plane, and we wouldn't charge anyone to use it. I made sure that use of the plane was controlled by Miss Bowen, my trusted personal assistant, and by nobody else. When Miss Bowen retired, that power was handed over to her successor Janice Darrah. The reason I gave Miss Bowen the responsibility was that she was the only one who could tell me that I couldn't use the plane. She was a formidable woman. I remember once asking her whether the plane was available to go to New York the next day. When she responded that it wasn't available, I asked, "Where is it?" She said, "It's in the air on the way to Memphis. A piece of machinery in Arvida has broken down. The company that makes the part is in Memphis, and they said that they couldn't send a man up to Arvida to fix it for another week, so the plane is already on the way to Memphis to pick him up."

By acquiring an aircraft, we could also adjust the organization and run it more efficiently. We originally had a rolling mill expert for Canada, another one for the US, another for Britain, another for South America, for Japan, and so forth. With the help of the plane, we were able to reduce that number to one expert who was located in Germany. We made sure that no rolling mill investment anywhere in the world was approved unless he went to the location and confirmed that it was the right thing to do. Because of the bad rap that corporate planes inevitably get, a lot of companies that owned a plane didn't put their logo on it. I did the reverse. I put Alcan's logo on our plane. When we bought our Challenger 601, the first one that Canadair sold, we got it at a very good price. I refused to have it painted. After all, we were in the aluminum business, so why not show off the aluminum? I soon discovered that if you don't paint an airplane you have to apply a special polish for slipstream purposes, so we paid the extra money to have it polished. When I left Alcan the corporate planes were sold, reflecting a different management philosophy. Yet nobody can convince me that corporate jets are not efficient tools if used right. At the salaries they're paying C E O s these days, it's crazy to have them sitting around airport terminals for hours at a time. There's no point having an airplane if you're not using it at least 700 or 800 hours a year, and you can't do that if you're only using it to cart the C E O around. It needs to be made available to anybody in the company who can argue that it makes business sense to do so. Many corporations may not own their own jets anymore but aircraft-sharing businesses run by firms like NetJets have grown exponentially, so the message has got across.

I have always been fascinated by airplanes, so it was a natural for me to serve on the board of Canadair when it was owned by the Canadian government. Among the many memorable people I met while on that board was James B. Taylor III, a master corporate jet salesman, who joined Canadair in the late 1970s just as the Challenger business jet program was beginning to take shape. Canadair was considering a design drawn up by Bill Lear of Learjet fame, and, like his earlier planes, it was sporty and cigar shaped. Knowing his potential customers for the Challenger, Jim Taylor insisted on a passenger cabin that was wider and higher than originally envisaged. It was the right decision, not just for the Challenger, as it allowed Bombardier, which eventually bought Canadair, to develop the Challenger into the highly lucrative Canadair Regional Jet.

Like any great salesman, Jim Taylor had an inexhaustible repertoire of business jet stories and anecdotes. "If you like bus travel, then use the commercial airlines," he used to remind his prospects. A favourite story of his concerned a businessman who was checking in at La Guardia airport in New York for a flight to Dallas and tells the ticket agent, "Listen carefully. I have three bags with me. I want one to go to Chicago, the second to go to Los Angeles, and the third to come with me to Dallas." The ticket agent responds, "I'm very sorry sir, we can't do that. We can only accept bags that will go with you to Dallas." To which the businessman replies, "I don't understand why you can't do that. You managed to do it when I flew with you last week."

When Jim was still selling the French-made Falcon business jet, before he joined Canadair, he was in Los Angeles and had a prospective buyer to whom he offered a demo flight to Las Vegas and back to show off the jet. The client accepted, and, as the two took off from LA, Jim quickly realized that his prospect had little interest in the technical specs of the plane, so he switched to general topics. On arriving in Las Vegas, the stairs went down and the red carpet was unrolled, but the prospect stayed in his seat. Then a tall and well-endowed young woman, probably a showgirl, came on board and greeted the prospect warmly. "Okay Jim," he told Taylor. "She fits, so I'll buy it."

As part of the hunt for new customers, I used to travel to Czechoslovakia to peddle ingot. The volumes they were taking may not have been huge, but the Czechs had hard currency and every sale helped. It was the height of the Cold War, and I hated every minute of those sales trips. Prague was a beautiful city, but it had a huge, wet Communist blanket smothering it. There were no smiles, no life, and we were constantly being followed by the secret police. The routine was the same for every trip. I would go to Zurich and pick up one of the Alcan people from our Zurich office, a man who was called Herr Schmidt. Why Zurich? We were always negotiating contracts for aluminum in Prague, and, because we were behind the Iron Curtain and knew our phones were being bugged, the only way to have secret conversations with the outside world was to speak in the Swiss German dialect, which we knew the Czech spies would never understand. Herr Schmidt was great fun. We were usually in Prague for a week, and every morning he would go to the newsstand just outside the hotel and mischie-vously ask for a copy of the *Neue Zuericher Zeitung*, Switzerland's leading daily newspaper. "Sorry, it didn't come in this morning," the fellow at the newsstand would inevitably reply. Of course, the paper never did come.

The man at the state metal import agency with whom we dealt was a Czech who did not appear to be a convinced Communist but had gone along with the regime to survive. I once asked him why he was willing to spend five days haggling with us simply to get a quarter of a cent discount off of the price of a pound of alu-minum. His answer was simple, "Because if I succeed, I get a big-ger apartment." Even in the heart of the Soviet Bloc they were using capitalist-like incentives to motivate managers. It's human nature, I guess. Another incentive used consistently by the Czechs with their business associates was alcohol. They would ply you with gallons of vodka. As for the food, it was very dreary except for the national dish of goose liver and dumplings, with thick gravy, which was delicious if a little rich.

After one of these sales trips to Prague, I was asked to take the Czech Ambassador to Canada for a visit to Arvida to show him our installations. The ambassador was a history professor by train-ing who had bought heavily into the Communist system. Those were the days when all that the *nomenklatura* in Communist countries like Czechoslovakia did was give you statistical evidence of the great progress they were making – exciting stuff like figures on the production of pig iron or tractors. When I took this man to Arvida, I actually spent very little time showing him around the smelters and other industrial facilities. I figured I didn't have to impress him with the number of megawatts produced by our dams or the monthly output for aluminum ingots. Instead, we visited the homes of workers; I just knocked on doors to show him the lifestyle of ordinary people in a prosperous, non-Communist country. One day, in an attempt to make conversation over lunch, I mentioned how much I had grown to love goose liver and dump-lings during my visits to Prague. "Oh yes, that is our national dish," the ambassador said. I then noted that, despite its delicacy, goose liver was a bit fattening. He agreed, "Yes, our population is

10,000 metric tons overweight." That's Communist statistics for you! All I can say is that those dreary visits to Czechoslovakia in the 1950s made me appreciate everything we had in Canada. At the end of the week, when the door would close on the Swissair DC-3 at Prague airport for the flight back to Zurich, I always breathed a sigh of relief.

Our need to find new markets for aluminum increasingly lent the company a certain missionary zeal. At times, it seemed as if there wasn't a country where we wouldn't consider setting up an extrusion plant or a joint venture to market aluminum. We just felt we owed it to the natives to be there and deliver the good news about aluminum, like Jesuits spreading the word of Christ. The other producers did this as well, but for us there was the simple fact that we had a home market that could only use 10 or 15 per cent of the aluminum we produced. It had been Edward K. Davis's plan right from the beginning for Alcan to take on the whole world. His older brother was quite happy to stick mostly to the United States, and he gave the rest of the world to his kid brother. So it should be no surprise that when our proselytizing was at its most extensive, Alcan was operating in twelve countries in Africa.

The product of choice in Africa was corrugated aluminum roofing. At one time, we had a salesman in Ghana with an original approach. He used to go around to all the villages and trundle about with him two portable structures each about the size of an outdoor privy. One would have a rusted corrugated steel roof and the other a shiny Alcan aluminum roof. He would install a big thermometer inside each. He'd leave the two structures in the village square in the blazing West African sun, and people would come around and marvel at the lower temperature in the aluminum-topped hut. These were simple sales methods, which were highly effective, but, considering the cost of doing business in that part of the world, it was all very expensive and not very profitable. What I figured at one point was that the overhead costs of being everywhere were prohibitive. Overhead will kill you if you try to take on the whole world at once. In the end, we pulled out of Africa as we withdrew from marginal markets around the world.

4

"Je me souviens"

Alcan's Québécois Heart

Growing up in Montreal prior to the Second World War, it wasn't hard for English Canadians to ignore the reality of French Canada. The English and French worlds were quite separate, divided not just by language but also by religion, education, and social class. Montreal was a much more anglophone town then than now, not just because of the economic dominance of its elite but also because of the demographic weight of the English-speaking community at the time.

Although it might have been easy to live in Montreal while ignoring French Canada, its culture and history, that was not the way I was raised. My first memories of recognizing the difference that is Quebec probably came from my mother. Fern used to say to me, "I don't understand why people say that Montcalm wasn't a great general. He won every battle he fought except for the last one when he was sick and greatly outnumbered." From the very beginning my mother had French Canadian friends. Granted, they spoke to her in English because her French wasn't very good, but she saw no difference between French Canadians and anybody else. Fern's mother was Catholic, and despite her father's efforts to give her a good Protestant upbringing, my mother quite liked Catholicism. In fact, in later life she was enamoured with the rites of the highest possible High Church Anglicanism where religion and pageantry are closely intertwined. She always said that the High Anglicans had stolen the art of religious ceremony from the

Roman Catholic Church. The upshot of all this was that when I
first heard the phrase "two solitudes," to indicate the mutual isola-
tion of English and French Canadians, I remember being angry
and thinking it was a lot of nonsense because I had grown up in an
atmosphere where there were no such solitudes.

Later in life, I did form the opinion that there was a problem, a
problem caused by what I would call the partially well-founded
superiority complex of the anglophone community versus the
partially well-founded inferiority complex of the francophone
community. In both cases, these were deep-rooted complexes that
related to history and to each community's educational and social
background. In thinking about this partially well-founded inferiority complex among francophones, I always look back to the
period of almost one hundred years that elapsed between the
British Conquest of New France in 1760 and the arrival in Quebec
City of the French corvette La Capricieuse in 1855. During that
century not a single vessel sailed between France and Canada.
Nothing explains more dramatically France's abandonment of its
former colony and its inhabitants than this fact of history, which
illustrates why that vacuum was so easily filled by the largely
agrarian and conservative Catholic Church. With its iron grip on
a small and isolated society, the Church dominated Quebec well
into the twentieth century, with serious consequences for its economic and social development. As I look back on my life, what
pleases me about Canada as much as anything else is that both
these so-called partially well-founded complexes have been erased.
It's true that there are still scraps of the old feuds left in both
the anglophone and francophone societies, but they are simply
remnants.

When the winds of change blew through Quebec in the twentieth century, Alcan became a major catalyst for development, particularly in the aptly named Royaume du Saguenay, the Kingdom
of the Saguenay. Along with the pulp and paper industry, in the
space of a few short decades Alcan transformed the Saguenay from
a sparsely populated region dominated by agriculture and forestry
to an industrial powerhouse. And, more remarkable still, this

company, with its US origins and multinational ambitions, did so while retaining a remarkably positive rapport with the Quebec public, particularly in the Saguenay. Over the years, I've often been asked why Alcan seemed to have such smooth relations with successive Quebec governments whatever their political stripe. While other large Canadian companies based in Montreal would occasionally incur the wrath of Quebec nationalists and be accused of lacking sensitivity to the French fact or of treating the province like a colony, Alcan seemed to escape that kind of opprobrium. As a company, we always worked hard to have the best community relations possible, whether we were operating in Jamaica or Guinea or Australia. In the case of Quebec I really think that our understanding and appreciation of the province and its people had been imbued in the Alcan culture from its early days and so became part of the company's DNA.

In 1929 when R.E. Powell was sent to Canada from Pittsburgh to run Alcan's growing aluminum business, he did things from the start that no English Canadian would ever have thought of doing. Rip Powell was no Francophile with a literature degree from the Sorbonne – he was an American from the Midwest, a man with an unfinished degree from Monmouth College who spoke little more than *merci* or *bonjour*. But, he was a brilliant salesman, businessman, and pragmatist who recognized that if Alcan was going to be based in Quebec, smelting aluminum with the province's abundant hydroelectric power, it should be seen above all as a loyal and committed corporate citizen. That meant embracing Quebec's language and culture, rather than ignoring it or wishing it away as was too often the case with the Anglo-Canadian business establishment. Soon after arriving in Montreal, Powell discovered that Alcan's legal head office was in Toronto because the law firm that had created the company was from Toronto. So he moved the head office to Montreal where operations were already centred. It was a symbolic gesture that still resonates many decades later.

Then Rip Powell made what was a daring move in the prewar Montreal business establishment where the lines between English and French were more sharply drawn than they are today. He

joined the Laval-sur-le-Lac Golf Club, the leading French Canadian
club and one that no English Canadian would have thought of
being part of at the time. He also became a member of the
Club Saint-Denis, Montreal's leading French Canadian businessmen's club. Mr Powell began hiring French Canadians and put
them in leading jobs at Alcan in the 1930s, top-grade men like
Paul Leman, Paul LaRoque, and Claude Beaubien. It was a revolutionary idea. As late as 1963, Donald Gordon, the controversial
president of Canadian National Railway, said publicly that the
state-owned railway didn't have any French Canadian vice presidents because it couldn't find any who were competent to do the
job. It set off a wave of nationalist protests against C N and Gordon
who was burned in effigy.

Alcan never encountered the kind of public enmity that other
big Anglo-Canadian companies did in Quebec. Rip Powell simply
accepted Quebec reality in a way that came naturally to him as
an American but wouldn't have been imaginable at the time to
Canadian anglophones, who looked at French Canada and saw a
society dominated by professions like law, medicine, and the clergy
with scant interest in the world of business and commerce. Rip
Powell saw no problem in promoting the use of French at Alcan
long before it was required by Quebec legislation. It was a recogni-
tion that was mutual. In 1949, Mr Powell was awarded an honorary doctorate by Laval University in Quebec City; it was an honour
that was unusual at the time for an anglo businessman. It's a tradition that continues to our day, even though ownership of Alcan
has passed to Rio Tinto, the Anglo-Australian resource giant. The
current C E O of Rio Tinto Alcan, the parent's aluminum subsidiary, is Jacynthe Côté, a native of the Saguenay who began her
career at Alcan as a process analyst at the Vaudreuil alumina refinery near Arvida and made a rapid ascent through company ranks
in Canada and Europe.

Ms Côté followed a well-trod path for francophone executives at
Alcan, spurred by a distinctive spirit of adventure. One of my tasks
at the company was to periodically ask people to uproot themselves and their families for a transfer to one of the far-flung parts

of the world where Alcan had operations. I don't think I ever had a francophone refuse a move, even to Africa and other difficult places to live. Sometimes I would ask, "Don't you want to consult your spouse first?" And the response would be, "Oh no, she'll go." When it came to Americans, you could get them to take one posting abroad after they left college, but generally speaking they weren't much interested in going elsewhere thereafter. English Canadians were a bit picky, but the Swiss, Scandinavians, Australians, and, above all, francophone Canadians were pretty much prepared to go anywhere. Again, I explain this through a bit of history. The voyageurs, the rugged types who would take off in canoes for two years and who opened up the West to the fur trade, were mostly French Canadians. They had the kind of sense of adventure that is very important in a global business. If you don't have a sense of spirit of discovery, it's very hard to get yourself to leave home and beat a path in search of business. One of the suggestions that I've made over the years to various Quebec premiers, so far to no avail, is that Quebec should celebrate that sense of adventure and erase any lingering sense of inferiority. A first step would be to change Quebec's license plates, which currently have the motto "Je me souviens" (I remember). Not exactly a forward-looking statement. Instead of "Je me souviens," we should have license plates that say "Allons-y" (Let's go). All I get back when I make the suggestion is a smile, but obviously nothing is ever going to be done about it. That's unfortunate.

More than thirty-five years after the event, it's hard to underestimate the convulsion felt in Canada and particularly in Quebec when René Lévesque and his separatist Parti Québécois came to power in November of 1976. For many English Canadians in Montreal, who had gone through the trauma of the October Crisis in 1970 and increasingly restrictive French language legislation, the prospect of an independent Quebec was just too much for them to contemplate. Many individuals and businesses decided to vote with their feet and began abandoning Montreal for Toronto. Quebec independence didn't really make much sense to outsiders either. Within days of the election of the P Q government, one of my American friends who had been studying Quebec wrote me a note that said, "What is sovereignty-association? Isn't that what Quebec already has?" I thought that was a very perceptive remark. While Quebecers may be adventuresome, they also wanted the security of continued association with Canada, a foot in both camps. Many years later, I would tell my friends on the board of Montreal's Jewish General Hospital, who wanted to remain a McGill teaching hospital but didn't want to be part of the merger of other leading English-language hospitals into the McGill University Health Centre, that what they were actually looking for was René Lévesque's concept – a form of sovereignty-association.

The oil shock of 1973 once again brought home to Alcan the value of its hydroelectric assets in Canada. It was clear that the days of smelting aluminum using electricity produced with cheap oil were over, and the advantage would swing to producers like Alcan. Already in 1974, Nathanael Davis told Alcan's annual meeting that, "the importance of the energy cost factor appears to have returned to the fore and Alcan believes that the time has arrived when it can undertake a systematic, medium-term program of expansion and modernization of its Canadian smelting facilities." The goal was to start construction of a new smelter in the Saguenay with completion in 1977. A 2,300-acre site was purchased near Ville de La Baie, about thirty kilometres from Arvida, and the project was dubbed the Grande-Baie smelter, but the oil spike sparked a recession, and the decision was delayed.

Yet the economic arguments in favour of a new Saguenay smelter were overwhelming, and the project was revived as soon as the prospect of an improved economic outlook became apparent. Alcan's hydroelectric facilities were producing more power than we could consume in our own plants, and the surplus was being sold to third parties, mainly Hydro-Québec, at low returns. In addition, because of obsolete smelting technology, much of it dating from the 1930s and 1940s, we were using too much electricity to make each ton of aluminum. In fact, Alcan was often criticized by the investment community for wasting its power-cost advantage through inefficiency in our smelters, particularly in Quebec. We estimated that we could increase our Quebec metal output by sixty per cent with the same amount of power, if we only modernized our smelting network. And, the power advantage that flowed from ownership of the dams was substantial. We estimated that the cost of power for a new smelter at La Baie would be just over three cents per pound of aluminum, compared with eleven cents for a new US smelter. In the previous decade, the international consumption of primary aluminum had grown at a staggering rate of almost nine per cent per annum, and even if that growth rate were to slow down, more metal was sure to be needed.

There was also concern that the company's obsolete smelters and inefficient use of its hydroelectric power would attract increased attention from organized labour and the Quebec government, particularly because of less-than-optimal working conditions at the old smelters and air pollution issues. Alcan's hydro assets had been left alone when the Quebec government nationalized most of the province's private power producers in the early 1960s, but there were periodic political rumblings that Hydro-Québec should buy out Alcan's power assets as well, which would have made our operations in the province a lot less attractive.

All of this came to a head in 1976, just a year after I had been appointed president of Aluminum Co. of Canada, Alcan's main operating subsidiary. I guess we all have a time in our lives when we experience what Queen Elizabeth II so aptly referred to as an *annus horribilis*, an awful year we'd all rather forget. For the Queen it was 1992, the year that her children Charles, Anne, and Andrew, all split from their spouses, in often-humiliating circumstances, and, to cap it off, the year ended with a devastating fire at Windsor Castle. For me, my *annus horribilis* was 1976, the year Alcan was rocked by a series of long and bitter strikes that closed down much of our Canadian smelting operations, costing the company tens of millions in lost profit and setting back the state of labour relations at the company for years. The context was one of rampant inflation, which the Canadian government was attempting to reduce through wage and price controls, a situation exacerbated in Quebec by a social ferment that climaxed with the election of the separatist Parti Québécois that autumn.

As far as the Saguenay strike is concerned, I always said that it was a matrimonial dispute. It took two of us to cause the strike. I never said that the strike was just the union's fault. Productivity in our Canadian smelters had fallen to disturbingly low levels, off by between 12 and 17 per cent from just five years earlier. In Arvida, we estimated that we would need an extra 487 employees simply to operate at the smelter's rated capacity and produce 9,000 tons less than in 1972. Sloppy behaviour had crept into the Quebec smelters, indicating a startling lack of common sense and self-discipline. There were incidents of workers throwing Pepsi bottles into the pots, which was very dangerous and could have caused explosions. As we entered negotiations, we were pretty rigid, and the union had frankly been spoiled a bit. It's true that there would not have been a strike if I had looked the other way, but I could not condone what I considered to be irresponsible behaviour. When the Saguenay strike dragged on for five-and-a-half months, the press tried to bait me into saying that the union was being unreasonable. But, I kept repeating that it was essentially a marriage tiff in which both parties were to blame, and both parties would be happy when it was over.

The union representing most of the 7,200 workers in the Saguenay seemed in no rush to sign a new agreement to replace the one that was coming to an end on 31 May. We decided that we wouldn't be held to ransom and instituted a policy of no contract, no work. On 31 May, we sent a letter to all employees insisting that we could not continue operating without a valid agreement. The next day, we announced we were shutting down two potlines at Arvida and laying off one hundred workers. The union objected, but we stuck to our guns and ordered the closing of two more lines plus other facilities, this time affecting 700 employees. At 7:30 on the morning of 3 June, the provincial labour conciliator told us the union had delivered an ultimatum. Either we agreed to the union's negotiating timetable within ten minutes or they were walking out. At 8 a.m., the real nightmare began.

At an aluminum smelter a sudden, unplanned shutdown is unthinkable. Shutting down any big industrial process is a sensitive thing to be done slowly, deliberately, and in stages. In aluminum smelting, that's even more essential. If power is suddenly cut to the giant pots, the molten metal in the electrolyte bath will freeze up, causing massive equipment damage. Before production can resume, the solidified aluminum must be removed from inside every pot, usually with a jackhammer. At Arvida the employees basically abandoned ship and sabotaged the main switching station, causing the pots to seize up and inflicting damage we estimated at $25 million. A similar situation reigned at Beauharnois and Isle Maligne.

What's worse, we experienced problems at the Kitimat smelter in British Columbia at the same time. There, the workers, members of an independent union, staged a wildcat strike, insisting that Alcan reopen a collective agreement that we had signed with them only months before. The workers were upset that the federal Anti-Inflation Board had okayed a higher wage settlement for B C pulp and paper workers. Most of the unionized workers at Kitimat walked out, but the power supply was uninterrupted and we were able to keep the smelter operating with a cadre of management personnel and workers who defied their own union to stay on the job. The strikers blocked road access to the smelter, so the only way to keep the plant provided with men and supplies was by helicopter, seaplane, or boat. Besieged in the smelter, they worked day and night to keep it operating. Aiding this heroic effort was a phalanx of 180 engineers and foremen from the idled Quebec plants whom we flew across the country to Kitimat to help out their colleagues. These managers and workers worked two six-hour shifts a day and caught sleep when and where they could, trapped in the smelter. But nobody complained, although lots of generous overtime payments didn't hurt their morale.

Things were clearly out of hand. Within the space of a couple of days, we had lost two-thirds of the output of our Canadian smelters, leaving only 315,000 tons still in operation out of annual capacity of more than one million tons. And, much of that capacity had been shut down in a brutal fashion. The situation in the Saguenay continued to spin out of control through much of the summer. The provincial police were preoccupied with helping secure the Summer Olympic sites in Montreal. Strikers attacked management staying at a local hotel, using threats and even their fists against Alcan managers and the company's lawyer. Molotov cocktails were launched outside the Vaudreuil alumina refinery. In early September, a group of fifty vandals broke into the Arvida smelter and used chains to break power cables and drain electric transformers of their oil, causing even more damage. It was clear to us that the raid had been carefully planned. More than one hundred cars had been used to block access roads to the plant.

As the strike continued, everybody was becoming fed up and exhausted. The union was sick of it. The company was sick of it. The wives were sick of it. Then, Quebec Provincial Court Chief Justice Alan Gold was named a mediator in the case. He was a wonderful guy and a veteran mediator who managed to solve some of the most contentious labour disputes in the country, involving longshoremen and postal workers, while still maintaining the respect of both sides.

I had the pleasure of working with Judge Gold on the board of McGill University, where he was the chairman for a time. He was a marvellous leader. I can remember one board meeting in the 1960s, at the height of the student protest movement, when the door opened and twelve students, each carrying a placard, marched into the boardroom. They sat at the back of the room and held up their placards. Judge Gold turned to them and said calmly, "Now, we're pleased to have you students here, but we won't have placards, so please put them down." All the placards quietly came down except for the one held by the leader of the group who still held his high in an act of defiance. Judge Gold addressed him directly, "You know, I have the power to have you removed from this room, but if I do that not only might you not hear something that you should hear but we might not hear something that we should hear. I would much prefer if you put down the placard and stayed here with us, rather than have you removed." The guy put his placard down and the tension dissipated. Alan Gold really had the wisdom of Solomon. So you can imagine my relief at seeing him named to mediate this terrible dispute.

When Judge Gold met the two sides, he said, "Gentlemen, the fact is, I've promised my wife to take her to Florida. Don't worry. I'll be back in two weeks, and I'll see you then." Both sides were shocked and horrified, which was no doubt the kind of reaction Judge Gold had hoped for. He wanted both sides to cool down and contemplate their positions. Two weeks later, as promised, the judge returned to Montreal and called me and Roger Phillips, who was running our Canadian smelting arm, to his chambers at the courthouse at 3 p.m. I suggested to Roger that he listen hard and talk little. That was something that Roger found difficult to do, and he was soon criticizing the union for being unreasonable.

Judge Gold turned to us and replied, "Let me tell you a story. A wise rabbi was visited one day in his office by a male member of his congregation who complained about the behaviour of his wife, the fact that she was playing bridge all the time, and neglecting the children. The rabbi responded, 'You are right. I must do something about your wife.' The next day, the wife arrived at the rabbi's office and proceeded to complain about her husband, that he was drinking and chasing women and failing in his obligations. 'You are right. I must do something about your husband.' At that point, the rabbi's assistant, who had been there for both visits, said, 'Yesterday you said that he was right, and today you are saying that she is right. They can't both be right.' The rabbi looked at his assistant and said, 'you're right'!" At which point, Judge Gold told Roger and me, "Do I make my point? I am not here to say who is right and who is wrong. I am here to settle this strike."

Judge Gold then looked me in the eye and said, "I need more money to settle the dispute." I responded that I couldn't give him more money. Only Louis Mongrain could give him more money.

Louis was the line manager in Arvida negotiating with the workers. He had no idea I had just handed him the freedom to up Alcan's offer.

Gold thanked us, and we left. That same evening he jumped on a Quebecair flight to Bagotville, arrived in nearby Jonquière, and checked into a hotel. He called Mongrain and asked him to come over. When Mongrain arrived, Gold took out a long sheaf of paper and started writing. He asked Mongrain to stand just behind him and told him he was going to write up the terms of the proposed contract. Gold told Mongrain that if he objected to any clause he should tap him on the shoulder. Mongrain never did, and that's how we got the settlement, which, nevertheless, took another excruciating period before it was approved by the union membership. The new pact was finally okayed by a union vote on 15 November. A separate strike dragged on at Shawinigan until January of 1977, but by then, thankfully, my *annus horribilis* had ended.

I learned a few lessons from this strike, including one about timing. It's easy to get people to start a strike in the warm summer months, when the weather is good, there's fishing to be done and school is out, but it becomes a lot more difficult to keep up the enthusiasm as time goes by. And, because of the complications in shutting down and restarting an aluminum smelter, if you have a strike or a lockout and it lasts more than twenty-four hours, chances are that it will last for twenty-four weeks.

As it turns out, the vote that ended the strike in the Saguenay took place on another day that was to have huge significance, 15 November 1976. That day René Lévesque's Parti Québécois was elected as Quebec's provincial government, promising to hold a referendum on separation for the province, which they preferred to call sovereignty-association. You can well imagine the consternation of the Alcan board of directors when they met in Brazil in April of 1977, and I told them I wanted to build a new $500 million smelter in Quebec and put it in the Saguenay. For me, the justification for the Grande-Baie smelter was overwhelming. We knew that we were going to need more aluminum, it was the right time from a business point of view to build, and we had the power available from our own hydroelectric facilities. But, with the wounds of the strike still not healed and Quebec threatening to wrest itself from the Canadian federation, the directors told me that I was nuts. It wasn't the time to make such a massive investment in Quebec, with a newly elected provincial government dedicated to breaking up Canada. My response was an attempt to be calming and get them to take the long view. "Look, this is only one of ten or fifteen governments that the province of Quebec will have during the lifetime of this new smelter," I told them. Finally one of the directors said, "If we approve your building a new smelter in the Saguenay at this time, you must get us a letter from Mr Lévesque written in his own blood saying that nothing will happen to this investment." I replied that the letter would be easy to obtain but not worth much. The next government would ignore it. Rather, I would safeguard the new investment by having it first announced by the mayor of La Baie. Lévesque was desperate to keep a modicum of credibility with the business community, particularly with a company like Alcan, so I knew he wasn't about to reopen the issue of nationalizing Alcan's hydroelectric facilities. He had too many other battles to fight, including his plan to buy a stake in the province's then-thriving asbestos mining industry. However, we did manage to secure an agreement with Quebec on the long-term indexed tax policy for private power generation, which provided us with increased certainty for the future of our investment.

I convinced the board to push ahead with Grande-Baie, though many of the directors thought it was an unwise idea. They saw ghosts under every bed when it came to Quebec. The next challenge became one of optics – how to announce this huge investment without appearing to be part of a corporate fan club for the separatists and at the same time not getting enmeshed in the increasingly bitter battle between federalists and the PQ over the future of Quebec. What I figured we had to do in order to depoliticize the issue to the greatest extent possible was to exclude both the federal and provincial governments. Instead, the announcement was made in May of 1977 by the mayor of La Baie where the smelter was to be built. I knew that the mayor would make sure that this huge investment for his community would not be scuttled by that bane of Canadian politics – a federal-provincial dispute. That approach worked like a charm. The announcement of the first 57,000-ton-a-year potline was followed in December of 1978 by a second phase and a year later of the third and final phase. It was Alcan's first new smelter in Canada in twenty-five years.

By the time the first phase of the smelter officially opened in September of 1981 (production began the previous December), I felt that my decision to go ahead with Grande-Baie had been vindicated, and it was time for a real celebration. More than 500 people, including politicians and business leaders from across the country, some flown in on charters from Toronto and Montreal, attended the official opening, and on the following day we flew up a planeload of financial analysts for a look-see. The heat and foul air of the Dickensian potrooms at the old Arvida smelter had been replaced by the spotless expanse of Grande-Baie's massive smelting halls where the air was clear and employees scarce, reflecting the efficiencies we had gained with new technology.

What made the smelter even more attractive to the financial analysts was the fact that we had managed to keep the Grande-Baie facility nonunion by proving to Quebec labour authorities that the smelter added capacity to the Alcan system rather than replacing old facilities, and thereby involved no displacement of existing workers. We purposely kept all other installations unaffected. When we advertised for 800 new jobs at the Grande-Baie smelter, we got 21,000 applications! The nonunion environment proved attractive to both sides. Without the need to accept hidebound rules that had emerged from decades of bureaucratic collective agreements and the endless interpretations of labour lawyers and mediators, we could eliminate practices like bumping and layer upon layer of job classifications. When we started up Grande-Baie, I think there were only five pay classifications in the whole plant. You got paid not according to the classification you worked in but the number of job skills you possessed. If you qualified for all five classifications, you got paid the top rate. The employees loved this multiskilled approach because it eliminated much of the boredom that comes with industrial work. A Grande-Baie employee could run a crane on a Monday, work on a potline on a Tuesday, and then use his skills in the lab on a Wednesday. It created variety, and it encouraged teamwork. The problem with union rules is that they make work boring. More than thirty years later, Grande-Baie remains nonunion and employees have a high sense of job satisfaction.

In my remarks at the official opening, I called Grande-Baie, "a milestone, helping us to mark the point in history when we committed ourselves to take on the future and to modernize and rebuild our existing facilities in Quebec." By building a state-of-the-art smelter, I had a model that I could point out to politicians and investors alike as the way forward for Alcan. That was certainly the case with Premier Lévesque, who I knew could be a bit nasty at times but was also dead straight as a politician. In the early 1980s, when Alcan began to set up serious long-term plans to modernize its smelting capacity in Quebec, I asked the premier if he had ever been to Gary, Indiana, or Bethlehem, Pennsylvania. He hadn't. I suggested it would be worthwhile for him to see these one-industry towns whose steel mills had never been modernized so he could witness the decline and destruction that had resulted. I promised him that if Quebec were to extend Alcan's water rights on the Peribonca River, where we had major hydroelectric facilities, for a period of fifty years, Alcan would rebuild all of the old potlines in Quebec, replacing them with ultramodern clones of Grande-Baie, at an estimated cost of $3 billion. Alcan kept its word. In 1984, we announced construction of a new $1 billion smelter at Laterrière, which set off a massive rebuild of Alcan's smelting base in the province. Over the succeeding twenty-five years, Alcan built new, clean, energy-efficient smelters not only at Laterrière but at Alma as well and progressively shut down its older smelters. The Grande-Baie smelter also set off a wave of expansion by other aluminum producers in the province. New smelters were built at Sept-Îles, Bécancour, and Deschambault after Hydro-Québec signed long-term power supply contracts with several producers, and Reynolds Metals also expanded its big facility at Baie-Comeau. Alcoa, which had traditionally kept out of the smelting business in Canada since the split with Alcan in the 1920s, became a big presence, but it was hard for us at Alcan to object. We, more than anybody else, could hardly argue that Quebec wasn't a great place to make aluminum. And, there was just a trace of irony in that Alcoa decided to place its regional office in Montreal's Place Ville Marie, the aluminum-clad skyscraper where Alcan's head office spent twenty happy years.

Aluminum smelting is a hugely capital-intensive business that may create lots of construction jobs when new facilities are being built but not very many fulltime positions once a smelter is in operation. The desire for more jobs sparked a consistent drumbeat from politicians to do more in the way of secondary aluminum processing. I would repeat consistently that Quebec was a wonderful place to smelt aluminum but not an ideal place for a huge rolling mill that makes sheet for beer cans or a facility that bangs out aluminum wheels for cars. I would tell whoever would listen that, "the more you manufacture, the closer you have to be to your customers, and a big rolling mill doesn't really employ that many people in any case." The mantra of more manufacturing never let up, but we stood our ground, manufacturing what we could and no more, even when we were offered generous government subsidies.

Unlike other companies, Alcan never spent too much time cozying up to politicians. I always refused to take grants from governments, particularly those aimed at regional development, because you'd inevitably end up building plants in the wrong place simply because cash was being dangled in front of your nose. In the late 1980s, General Motors of Canada asked me to join their board. I told them I wasn't interested. They had just accepted a combined loan of $220 million from the federal and Quebec governments to finance a modernization of their auto assembly plant at Ste-Thérèse, north of Montreal. The governments agreed because otherwise GM said it would close the assembly plant, the only automotive facility of its kind in Quebec. Terms of the loan were about as generous as could be imagined – thirty years, interest free. I told GM that they could afford to finance their own plants and shouldn't be going to governments with cap in hand. Sure enough, GM took the cash but closed the plant in any case in 2002. The facility has since been demolished and replaced by a shopping mall, yet GM still owes the original principal to taxpayers. In the end, I always took the same approach as I.W. Killam did with taxes. Don't do the wrong thing for the right (grant) reason.

Although we did our utmost never to pick a fight with the provincial government, staying loyal to Quebec as a place to do business took patience at times. I remember this story from an Alcan employee in Kingston, Ontario whom we had brought to Montreal so we could offer him a job at head office. He was staying at the Queen Elizabeth Hotel, just across from Place Ville Marie, and went to the bar to have a drink. Who should he meet there but Jacques Parizeau, the PQ finance minister and a habitué of those kinds of establishments. When the Alcan man explained to Parizeau that he was an English Canadian from Kingston about to move to Montreal, Parizeau told him, "Stay in Kingston, we don't need you here in Quebec." Not much of a welcome mat. The employee was annoyed, to say the least, but he came anyway.

Lévesque was a more likable character, a totally self-confident guy. After he left office, he called one day and asked if he could come and visit Maison Alcan. I told him during his visit, "There are two things I like about you. In the first place, you contributed to the elimination of the two scorpions in a bottle situation in Canada. I also told him that he reminded me of the coach of a US college football team who lost twenty-one games in a row and said only, 'you can't win them all.' You lost twenty-one by-elections in a row for the Parti Québécois, and still you didn't change the rules."

In the 1980s, with the referendum defeated but the PQ still in power, the big provincial pension-fund manager, Caisse de Dépôt et Placement du Québec, was actively accumulating the stock of Montreal-based companies, and Alcan was no exception. At one point, the Caisse had as much as ten per cent of Alcan's stock, creating an uncomfortable situation for us. We had to be civil with the Caisse, as with any shareholder, but we had no desire to have a representative of the government on our board. Once a year I

would invite Jean Campeau, the Caisse's president, to come to dinner at the fancy dining room at Maison Alcan. Mr Campeau was a
low-key fellow, who was pleasant enough but seemed to be taking
orders from Mr Parizeau, the finance minister. Mr Campeau
would usually bring along another person from the Caisse as his
guest, and I would have my chief financial officer with me. After
dinner, when we were sitting around having a cigar, I would say,
"Mr Campeau, there are two reasons why I don't want to invite
you on to our board. The first one is that a lot of existing shareholders wouldn't like it, and, secondly, the Caisse can make a lot of
money by buying Alcan stock in the twenties and selling it in the
thirties and not be considered an insider. If you have representa-
tion on the board, you'd be an insider and couldn't do that anymore. So if you never ask me, I will never have to say no." And,
that's the way we left it. The Caisse never did get on to Alcan's
board, and relations with them and their political masters in the
Quebec government remained cordial. I'm convinced that if Alcan
had not had a history of good relationships with Quebec, I wouldn't
have gotten away with that kind of brush-off.

While I prided myself on maintaining good relations with the
Quebec government throughout my career, I did make one large
faux pas. In 1977, just after deciding to go ahead with Grande-Baie,
we announced that Alcan was going to close its research and
development centre at Arvida and consolidate all R & D at our labs
in Kingston, Ontario. It was the logical thing to do. It would have
saved money to consolidate the operations, but it was a P R disas-
ter for Alcan in the region. The announcement was seen as cutting
out the heart and soul of the Saguenay. Everybody in the community, from union workers to politicians, had always argued for
more R & D and more secondary processing and Arvida's R & D
was the cornerstone they were hoping to build on. The protests
became so extensive that I went up to the Saguenay personally and
reversed the decision. Sometimes you simply have to admit your
mistakes and do the right thing. In this case, the long-term impact
on Alcan's reputation was negligible or nonexistent.

This history of well-cultivated relations with the Quebec government probably contributed a lot to the ease with which Rio Tinto got Quebec's blessing to take over Alcan in 2007, many years after I had left the company. I'm often asked why Premier Jean Charest never objected to the takeover the way Saskatchewan's Brad Wall did when he effectively killed the takeover of Potash Corp. a few years later. The comparison is apt. Potash Corp.'s would-be buyer, a big Australian resource concern, B H P Billiton, dealt with Mr Wall and other provincial politicians in a ham-handed way prompting a complaint to Prime Minister Harper in Ottawa, who closed down the deal under foreign investment rules. Nothing of this sort happened with Rio Tinto, and I think it's because Quebec respected Alcan's management and its board. When the Charest government asked Alcan's leadership its view, it was told that Alcan didn't want to be taken over through a hostile bid from Alcoa. Rio Tinto was a reasonable alternative and was offering a very attractive price. If it was good enough for Alcan management, then the Charest government figured it must be good enough for the people of Quebec, so no objection went forth to Ottawa.

In 2007, the night before Alcan's final board meeting as an independent company, I was asked to address the directors at a special dinner. I repeated something to them that I had said several times before. "There's an expression in Europe: 'Scratch an internationalist and you'll find a provincialist.' Scratch a company that does business in sixty countries around the world and you'll find a Québécois." I added, "If you'll pardon the expression, as long as water runs downhill, Alcan will always be Québécois." I fearlessly predict that, in some form or another, Alcan will reaffirm or give witness again to its Quebec roots, perhaps when Rio Tinto tires of its foray into aluminum and Alcan once again becomes an independent company.

Over my lifetime, as Quebec has matured and come into its own, it's clear that Montreal's economic role has changed. It is no longer the Montreal of St James Street and I.W. Killam, the era when Canada's economy was run by Montrealers and by corporations run from the city. That time has passed. As I wrote in an article in the Montreal *Gazette* in 1996, "we should not compete with Toronto for the head offices of purely Canadian businesses. Montreal is not the best place from which to run an enterprise that sells its products and services only in Canada." What Montreal should strive to do is become "the Geneva of the twenty-first century, the preferred city from which to run global enterprises, a magnet for young people who use the new technologies as a means of making their individual mark on the world stage. A French city that confidently welcomes all languages, religions, and cultures."

As I wrote then and still believe, Montreal has fabulous attributes, including a school system and society where people of different origins, francophone Canadians, "Wasp" anglophones, Jews, Ukrainians, Chinese, Haitians, and many others meet, study, and learn about each other. This provides internationally-minded business with a wonderful pool of employees who can be sent anywhere in the world on short notice, knowing how to behave and get along. But, to really succeed in the goal of becoming a latter-day Geneva, Montreal needs an inner peace that makes international capital comfortable with investing here. "For that to happen our politics can be lively, but they must never be nasty. Only we Quebecers can bring this about," I wrote at the time. "If we fail, our city will continue to decline to a point where it becomes a small regional town taking in the washing of other communities. If we succeed in achieving inner peace and if we use our energies and goodwill to make Montreal the leading French city in the world from which to manage global enterprises, our future is too exciting for words."

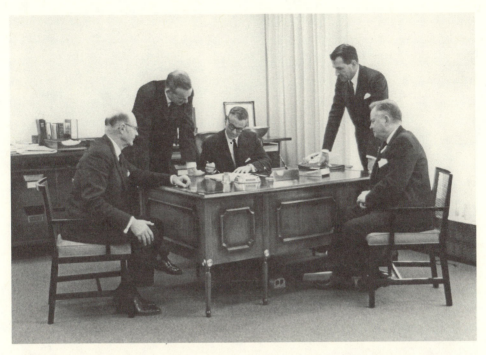

Competent, uncomplicated, and honest. Alcan Management Group, 1967: Scotty Bruce, Dana Bartholomew, Nathaniel Davis, and Mel Weigel. I was listening. (Courtesy of Rio Tinto Alcan)

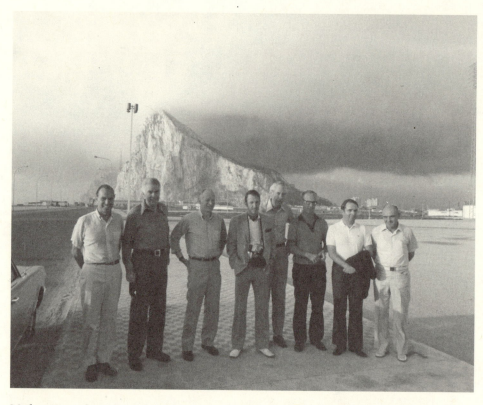

My happiest Alcan days with my exceptional area managers: Harold Corrigan, Eric Trigg, Eric West, John Clarkson, John Elton, Patrick Rich, and Jack Boetschi. I'm fourth from the left, with a camera. Gibraltar, 1975. (Courtesy of Rio Tinto Alcan)

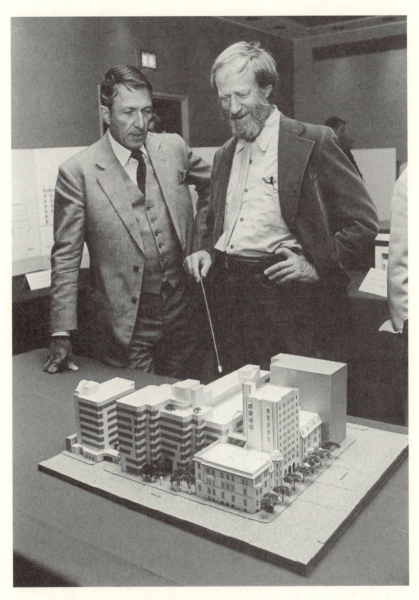

Ray Affleck was chosen to create Maison Alcan because of his nickname "Mr Sherbrooke Street." (Courtesy of Rio Tinto Alcan)

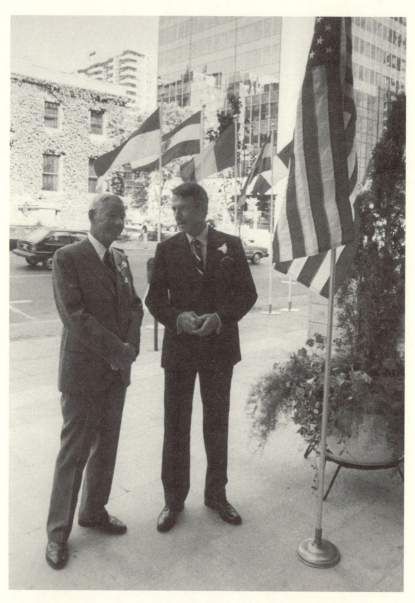

Inaugurating Maison Alcan with Nat Davis, 1983. It stopped people asking "Are we staying in Montreal?" (Courtesy of Rio Tinto Alcan)

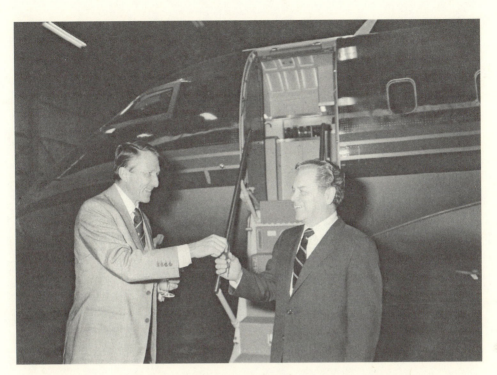

"It's your plane, and don't let anyone, including me, ask you to do with it what you're not in favour of." Handing Alcan Chief Pilot Lyle Hollinger keys to our new Challenger 601 in 1984. (Courtesy of Rio Tinto Alcan)

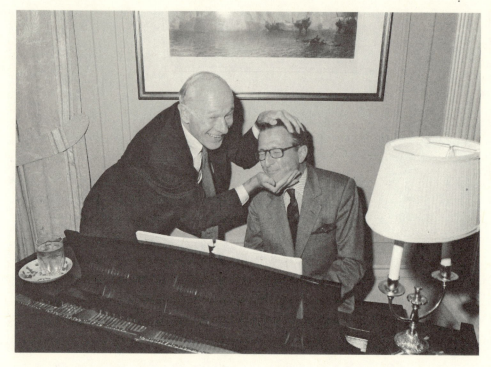

Eric West's retirement party, 1985. A special colleague. Guests were limited to ladies who had worked as his assistants over the years. (Courtesy of Rio Tinto Alcan)

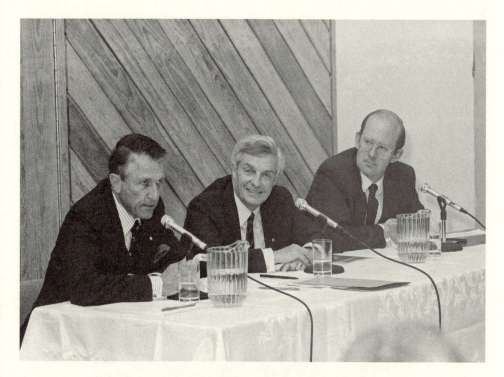

A rare entry into politics – talking Canada–US free trade with Alberta Premier Peter Lougheed and Canada's Deputy Chief Negotiator Gordon Ritchie, 1988. (Courtesy of Rio Tinto Alcan)

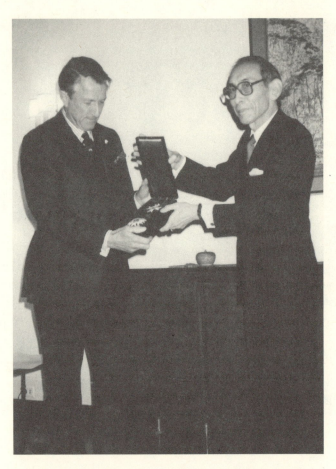

I received the Order of the Sacred Treasure from Yoshio Okawa, Japanese Ambassador to Canada, in 1987. (Courtesy of Rio Tinto Alcan)

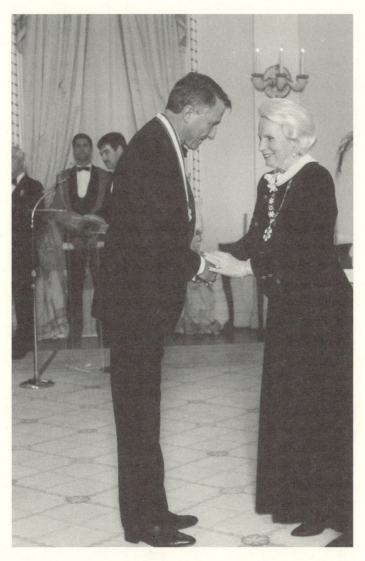

I was promoted to Companion of the Order of Canada by Governor
General Jeanne Sauve in 1988. (Courtesy of Rio Tinto Alcan)

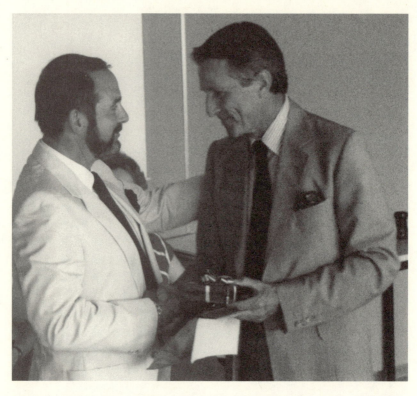

With the multi-talented Patrick Rich, 1984. (Courtesy of Rio Tinto Alcan)

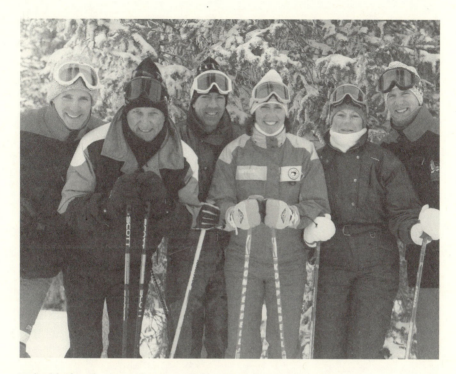

Valuable family time. Skiing in Colorado in 1989 with Mary and our children Andrew, Michael, Diane, and Mark.

5

"Dimension, Dimension, Dimension"

How Architecture Became a Passion

As a student, I never had much interest in architecture. Perhaps I took good architecture for granted. I couldn't draw, and I didn't want to become an architect. What awakened my interest in architecture and design were my postwar studies in Geneva that allowed me to travel across Europe and see some of the exquisite dimensions in the built landscape. We've all heard the expression "location, location, location" when discussing real estate. It's a factor you can't deny. I also like to refer to "dimension, dimension, dimension" when it comes to architecture. You can't deny that either. Good architectural design begins with the correct dimensions of a room or a foyer or an auditorium, and once those are set, the design is unchangeable. And dimension became something I began to look for in architecture and came to appreciate.

I got my first chance to test my developing interest in architecture in 1964, when I decided that the time had come to build a small house of our own in the country. As a wedding present, my father-in-law had given Mary a lovely piece of property on Lac Manitou, a picture-postcard lake near Ste-Agathe in the heart of the Laurentian Mountains cottage country north of Montreal. The tract of land was beautiful, but I didn't have much money to spend. Together with my brother-in-law, Tony Dobell, who was also building a small house on the same property, we chose a Montreal architect, René Welter. I soon discovered a truth that I've been conscious of ever since; the first thirty minutes that you spend with your architect are the most important thirty minutes. If you don't plant an idea in his mind in that first half hour, he'll develop one of his own, and the result will be a product of his conception rather than of yours. If you want to have any say in what happens, it's worth spending a lot of time thinking about what you're going to say to your architect in that first thirty minutes.

When I had my initial meeting with René, my suggestion to him was that in designing the house he should keep in mind that our family is an outdoor family and that we would really only be inside the house when we could not be outside. Therefore, it was important to have good views of the lake and the landscape around the house should be clearly visible from inside the house. The result is that all of the rooms, including bathrooms, were designed with floor-to-ceiling windows, and there is a glass panel between the roof of the house and the walls. Much of the outside is visible from inside!

The problem is that I didn't have much money to spend, and the first design exceeded my budget. As a compromise, we deducted one foot in every direction and went ahead. The total construction cost came to $57,000, which I was able to handle, but even today, forty-five years later, I look at that house and think how much better it would have been had we not reduced its dimensions by those twelve inches.

Before long, with that initial positive architectural experience in the country behind me, I began to think about what to do with our city house. When I moved back to Montreal in 1956, I had bought an old home on Westmount Avenue in Westmount. By 1970, we had lived there for fourteen years and had reached the point where we either had to spend major money on it or move, and we knew that in a few years the children would start moving out. About that time, the doorbell rang, and an old school friend of mine from Selwyn House, Edward Ballon, who had been living in Vancouver and was moving back to Montreal, was at the door. "I'd like to buy your house," he told me. Talk about happenstance intervening in my life once again. I said, "Okay, but you'll have to give me six months." We sold the house on Westmount Avenue and had six months to find a new place.

There were lots of houses on the market in Montreal at the time because of the political situation, something that was going to remain a factor for the following ten years at least. Mary started looking for a new place, but everything she was shown was either less house than we currently had at a higher price than we would be getting for ours, or the agent would say, "You'd better make up your mind fast because Mr Ballon is going to buy it." Well, Mr Ballon had already bought our house, so we knew that was a lot of nonsense. Months went by and we still couldn't find anything we liked. One day Mary and I were sitting at the table with the four kids and Andrew, who would have been about seventeen at the time and the least practical of the bunch, heard us talking and said, "What's wrong with this house?" I said, "Where have you been? We sold it four months ago, and we have to get out in two months." Suddenly aware of the urgency of the situation, Andrew piped up, "Oh, if we're looking for a place to live, why don't we buy that land on Clarke Avenue and build something?" I said, "Where on Clarke Avenue?" To which Andrew replied, "In the circle at the top of the street." I figured Andrew must have been dreaming. "There's no land for sale up there." Andrew was getting impatient. "Yes, there is. I just walked by with the dog, and there's a For Sale sign there."

With that, I jumped up from the table and ran up Clarke Avenue to a quiet cul-de-sac at the top of the street that I'd always loved, with its large stone houses and glorious views of the city and the river. It was a village within a village, with no through traffic yet close to downtown and to public transit. Sure, as Andrew had said, there was a lot with a For Sale sign. I called my agent and asked who the owner was. She told me that it was Alan McCall, an older man who had been president of Drummond McCall, a long-established steel and aluminum distribution business, and someone with whom I'd gone fishing in the past. He lived in a house two doors away and had bought this additional lot, which had been a garden for the neighbouring house, some years before, thinking that one day, when his house got too big, he'd build a smaller one there. In the meantime, Mr McCall had become more interested in living at his farm near Lachute, north of Montreal, and decided to put this single lot on the market. I called him and asked him if he'd be willing to sell. He said he would, but wondered about the timing of my plans. "If you build on it right away," McCall said, "I'll sell the land to you for what I paid for it several years ago, provided I can take one carload of rock off the property and take it up to Lachute." He had excellent taste. Sitting on the property was a trove of large black volcanic rocks that had been used to enhance the garden.

In the end, I got the lot for $22,000. Now to build a house. I decided to call up a Montreal architect named Max Roth, who had done some work for me at Alcan designing office space at our headquarters and had impressed me by managing to keep a lid on the subcontractors and being very careful with Alcan's money. He was a penny pincher. I told him that I wanted to build a house on the land, but I didn't have a whole lot to invest. After all, at that time I was a mid-level manager at Alcan, earning far from a fortune and supporting a wife and four children. "How much money have you got?" Max asked. "I can spend $160,000," I told him. Max designed the house, but when the construction bids came in they were much higher, at $192,000. Max was apologetic, admitting right off that the mistake was his. He thought he had designed a $160,000 house, but the contractors convinced him he had miscalculated. Max mulled it over and told me the problem could not be fixed simply by tweaking the original design. "There's no way I can take this same design and cut it down because, once you start taking a foot off of everything, your dimensions get all wrong." I immediately thought of my Lac Manitou experience! So Max agreed to go back to the drawing board and return with a second design for a smaller house. That time the bids came in at $160,000, almost to the penny.

Then I had to break some bad news to him. "Things aren't going well," I told him. "I don't have that $160,000 anymore." Max again put on his thinking cap and two weeks later called me back, disappointed but anxious to salvage the situation. "I don't think we should quit," he said. I agreed. "Look, the first design was your mistake," I told Max. "The second mistake was mine because I told you that I had $160,000, and when you came in at that price, I got cold feet. Now let's take a third crack at it, but this time I'll pay for the design." The new budget was $140,000 for a house that was even smaller. Max wanted assurance that I was still serious, so he asked me to guarantee that I would go ahead and build if his third design came in at $140,000. I agreed, and when the construction bid came in at $138,000, I decided to give him the okay. Just six weeks into construction, I got a bill from the contractor for $1,500 of extras. It was a shock. I phoned Max and asked him what to do about it. "Meet me at the site at six o'clock this evening," he told me. "I'll have the contractor there, but let me do the talking. Don't say a word." I got up to the top of Clarke Avenue at six and the contractor was initially all smiles. Max, who looked like Christ on the cross, with a beard and a very sad gaze, got down to business. "Now, let me see the details of this $1,500," he told the contractor. The two guys started wrangling over every line. After about thirty minutes the contractor wasn't smiling anymore. Max had got the bill down to $500. Then he gave me a little wink and turned to the contractor. "By the way, one of these footings is eighteen inches off from where it should be." Indignant, the contractor raised his voice, "What do you mean?" and got out the drawings. As part of the foundation work they had sunk holes and filled them with concrete for the footings, and, sure enough, one of the footings wasn't where it was supposed to be. Max made it clear to the contractor in no uncertain terms that he'd have to make it right. "I have to move this footing eighteen inches?" blurted out the contractor, clearly irritated. "Good God, Max, do you know what that'll cost me?" Then Max gave me another wink, put his arm around the contractor and said, "You forget about the whole $1,500, and we'll accept the footing where it is."

Two years after my old friend knocked on the door and asked me if I wanted to sell our house, during which time we lived in a rented house downtown, we finally moved into the new place on Clarke Avenue. Then one day soon after, a $2,000 bill from the contractor arrived in the mail. Interesting, considering the fact that I had budgeted $140,000 for the house and the original construction bid had come in at $138,000. I phoned Max and asked him what I should do about it. "Pay it," he responded. I did, and in the end the house cost me exactly $140,000. Incidentally, I believe I am correct that serious inflation began in June 1972, the month we completed construction and moved in.

I have to admit that it's a house that was no beauty when viewed from the outside, but from the inside looking out, it was fantastic. The house had a stone front, like the more traditional homes on the street, and had lots of glass and aluminum. The style was what is now considered mid-century, lots of geometric lines with little ornamentation; a style that has gained new fans in recent years among the younger generation. We had to get rid of the peaked roof to save money, so it had a flat roof and looked as if it belonged in a newer suburb, like Town of Mount Royal or Hampstead, rather than in the Victorian environment of Westmount. It had a great little garden, with a stream and a pond, in the back. You entered the house on the ground level and climbed up one floor where there were four small bedrooms for the children and two bathrooms. The top floor included the master bedroom, kitchen, dining and living rooms. The idea of having the master suite on the top floor pleased us and actually is an interesting way of coping with the empty nest syndrome. Most couples figure that their house is too big when their children move out and leave the upstairs eerily empty, but people rarely move out of a house because of an empty downstairs.

We lived on Clarke Avenue for thirty-six years, but the multiple levels and many stairs became more problematic as time wore on. From the beginning, I had asked Max to include an elevator shaft that ran from the garage up to the top floor, but we never got around to installing an elevator. By 2007, Mary was having a lot of difficulty getting up and down the stairs, so I put the house on the market. Another house on the same circle, which was much older than ours but bigger, had sold for nearly $4 million, so I decided to ask $2.9 million for ours. I didn't get any takers. Finally, in the spring of 2008, I sold the house for $1.75 million to a fellow who renovated the place with the intent of flipping it. He claims he spent $500,000 on it and sold it for $2.1 million, so he didn't make any money on the venture.

As for me, that house ended up not being a bad investment. When I asked the Bank of Canada what $140,000 in 1972 was worth in 2008, they told me it came out to $863,000, so a sale price of $1.7 million meant I had a pretty good return on my investment. I guess paying that extra $2,000 to the contractor didn't break the bank in the end.

With two houses under my belt, I began to realize that I was developing a real interest in architecture. A couple of years later, in the early 1970s, a young architect named Peter Rose, who was a friend of my children, came to me with an unusual proposal. He wanted Alcan to become the sponsor of a series of architectural lectures that would feature some of the world's greatest architects. The public would be invited, and entrance to the lectures would be free. I asked Peter what sort of budget he was looking for, and to my amazement he came back with a figure of just $5,000. The idea intrigued me. It was just the kind of project that could make a contribution to the community and give Alcan the profile I thought it deserved.

When I asked Peter about a possible venue, he said he thought that McGill University might be willing to provide a hall. In line with our frugal budget for the series, we decided that these would be 6 p.m. events, and we'd treat participants to coffee and doughnuts afterward. It would deliberately be nothing fancy, proof to the public that even a big multinational company could watch its pennies. Thus in 1974 began eighteen years of the Alcan series of lectures in architecture. True, the budget climbed steadily every year, reaching around $30,000 by the end, but it was still pretty cheap, and it gave Alcan lots of excellent publicity. It also gave members of the public who attended a hugely worthwhile and enjoyable experience. Just a few of the names of those who participated will give you an idea of the international calibre of the architects, designers, and planners involved. They included Frank Gehry, Robert A.M. Stern, Cesar Pelli, Robert Venturi, Denise Scott Brown, and Peter Eisenman. Most of the lecturers were also good showmen, and the events always attracted a full house. The architectural world began to pay attention to Alcan because a lot of architects liked this series. In fact, it was so successful we extended the concept to Vancouver where we launched a partner series. I was made an honorary fellow of the Royal Architectural Institute of Canada, and I got the reputation of being not just a patron of architecture but somebody knowledgeable in the field, although I don't think I did much to deserve that.

Architecture started playing a bigger role in my professional life as well when in 1979 I embarked on construction of Maison Alcan, the company's innovative new headquarters in downtown Montreal. But, that time-consuming venture didn't prompt me to drop architecture from my private life. After all, building houses had become something of a habit. In 1981, I decided that the house at Lac Manitou that I had built in the 1960s needed a garage and maybe a large public room. I proposed to Peter Rose an unusual commission, asking him to design a garage that I could occasionally use as a banquet hall, adjacent to what I termed an "orangerie" after the French tradition of building light-filled conservatories to grow oranges and exotic plants. The successful result is probably the only garage on Lac Manitou with massive windows and a slate floor. When my son Andrew got married recently, we moved out the cars, the bikes and the spare tires and used it as a banquet hall for the wedding reception.

In building the garage and orangerie, money was not as much of a concern as it had been, so I didn't give Peter a strict budget the way I had with Max Roth so many years earlier. Maybe I should have, but, to be honest, I just went to town with this project. The original house had a foundation of solid rock, characteristic of its location atop the Laurentian Shield, so I thought that the new structure would also be sited on rock. But when the big excavator began to dig, it didn't find any rock. It just kept going deeper and deeper until it arrived at a level about twelve feet below where the garage floor was supposed to be. I asked Peter what we were going to do with that massive hole, and he said that it would give me a lot of storage space. I didn't find that to be a very appealing answer.

Then I woke up one morning at Manitou and said to myself, "Not storage space. I'm going to build myself a Japanese room under the garage," and I found a guy who worked at the C B C and whose hobby was making Japanese-style furniture and screens. What was strange is that this fellow had never actually been to Japan, but he had developed a keen appreciation of Japanese design and the skill with which to execute it. When you go below the garage today, you'll find a fairly sizeable classical Japanese room complete with a Japanese bath. It was an instant hit with my kids and grandchildren, who love staying there, sleeping on the tatami mats, and bathing in the Japanese way.

Though that garage cost a pretty penny, I wasn't finished with the Manitou house quite yet. In 1989, the year I left Alcan, at the far end of the garage, I decided to build what I call the house for two, a cozy place for my wife and myself to live in so that all the children and grandchildren could use the original house on the other side of the garage and leave us some privacy. I commissioned Peter Rose, who had designed the garage and the Japanese room, to design the new house, and he turned the project over to one of his younger associates, Nicholas Garrison. About the same time, Peter and Nick had a falling out. Nick did a fabulous job on the house for two. It's a small house, but it's got everything in it, and to me it's reminiscent of some of Frank Lloyd Wright's drawings. The rooms are not big, but the light is magnificent and the workmanship is lovely. It is an embodiment of another of my strongly-held views about architecture, which is that people tend to build houses that are too big and have too many rooms. I've never seen the appeal of massive houses with wings where nobody ever sets foot. I would rather have a small house, built carefully and tastefully. The walls and built-ins of the house for two are all crafted from beautiful maple veneer, and, once again, the views are to die for. Nick did a great job on the design, but Peter Rose has never seen the house. Every time I see Peter, who now teaches architecture at Harvard and still builds homes for wealthy clients, I ask him when he's going to come and visit, but he has not done so.

Then in 2003, I did something that a person my age should have long since grown out of. I fell in love with a piece of land in Georgia. In so doing, I broke one of my cardinal rules about secondary residences, which is that you should never own a place that's more than one-and-a-half hours away from your permanent home. Private real estate pays no cash dividends, but it does pay handsome psychological dividends. The catch is that the psychological dividends are declared weekly and must be picked up in person. Any week that you don't visit your privately-owned real estate is a week without the dividend. More than one-and-a-half hours away means fewer dividends.

Again, happenstance played a major role. Mary and I had driven down to visit her ailing brother who was living in Hilton Head, South Carolina. Having come all that way, we decided to spend an extra three or four days around Savannah, which was nearby, just over the border in Georgia. I called my eldest son, Michael, who at one time had done a lot of business with Gulfstream, which is based in Savannah, and asked him to suggest a nice place to stay. He replied, "I was just skiing with a guy who has what sounds like a fabulous place at the Ford Plantation. I'll call him and get him to book a room for you." Which he did. We thought we were going to a nice resort hotel, but when we arrived around nine o'clock at night at the appointed address outside of Savannah, all we could see was one white shack and a gate. I said to myself, "Boy, this place doesn't advertise much!" I was about to turn around and drive back into Savannah to find a place to stay when a man came running out saying, "Oh, Mr Culver, we're expecting you! Here's your room key. Do you know how to get there?" When I said that I didn't have a clue, he responded, "It's about a quarter of a mile. Keep to the right and don't take any left turns. When you get to the house, you'll find nobody there, but go upstairs. You're in room number one. Make yourselves at home."

When we got there, I turned to Mary and said that I'd never been to a hotel like this. It looked like a version of Tara from *Gone With The Wind*, sitting in the middle of a real estate development, one of those gated communities that had grown up in resort areas across the US South where people build their own homes facing a beach or a golf course. And sure enough, the next morning when we came downstairs to the dining room a real estate salesman was sitting there on the main floor waiting for us. His name was John Friday. "Welcome to the Ford Plantation. I'm going to show you around." I said, "John, we're here under false pretences. We thought this was a hotel. We have no interest whatsoever in buying anything. We always said that we wouldn't live in a compound and I've always said I wouldn't want to live at sea level. The chances of your interesting us in any property here is zero." These were two more Culver rules on secondary-home purchase that I was about to break.

It turns out that the Ford Plantation was indeed a real estate development but one with a fascinating history. Originally settled in the eighteenth century, it consists of 1,800 acres of land along the meandering Ogeechee River, in Georgia's Low Country about eighteen miles outside of Savannah. The plantation grew rice and later cotton but was devastated by the Civil War and its aftermath. In the 1920s, automaker Henry Ford bought the property and built a Greek revival style mansion on the shores of the river and turned it into his winter retreat, where he entertained family friends like the Vanderbilts, the Rockefellers, and the du Ponts. After the death of the Fords, the home and former plantation passed through several hands until 1998 when it was bought by an investor group that turned it into a private residential and golf community.

Like any good salesman, John Friday wasn't about to give up even though we said we weren't interested in buying. "Fair enough," he said. "You're going to be here for four days in any case. I'm going to spend the mornings showing you around and in the afternoons you can play golf. You'll have a good time." Mary and I patiently allowed the persistent Mr Friday to show us lot after lot, which were all fine pieces of land but not particularly evocative of the US South. Those plots could have been in suburban Milwaukee or Minneapolis. After two days of showing us around, he turned up again at the start of day three and finally admitted he wasn't getting anywhere with his standard offerings. "Today I'm going to show you something I'm not supposed to show you, a resale. It's a lot that was bought by a man in New York who now wants to sell it." It was half an acre along the shores of Lake Clara with gorgeous live oaks adorned with cascades of Spanish moss. Lake Clara, named after Henry Ford's wife, had been created in the 1700s when a berm was built into the Ogeechee River, diverting water to create ponds for growing rice.

I confided to Mary that if we ever were in the market, this was the kind of land we would want to buy. The fourth and final morning, trusty Mr Friday was there again, knowing that we were catching a plane and heading home at noon. "Before you go to the airport, let's go back out to that lot that you like," he proposed. We got there, and I did what I do at times. I shot from the hip. "What does the owner want for it?" When the salesman gave me the price, I told him straight, "I'm seventy-nine years old, and I've got no business buying anything, but I'll offer him 75 per cent of his price. But that's it. I'm not interested in anything else. We're flying back to Montreal, then driving up to our country house, and here's my cell phone number. Thanks for spending a lot of time with us in what was probably a useless exercise."

We arrived back in Montreal later in the day, and as we were driving up to the cottage, my cell phone rang. It was John Friday telling us that the owner had made a counter-offer. I got impatient, "John, I told you, it's not on." He responded, "It's my job to act as a link between the two of you, so I had to tell you what he said." I made it clear again that I wasn't interested. Another twenty miles and the phone rang. It was John trying again. "My client wants to split the difference." I was adamant. "Forget it," I told him. So we motored on, and then, just as we were turning into the driveway at Lac Manitou, the phone rang yet again. "Congratulations! You now own property on the Ford Plantation."

The seller had taken my lowball offer, and I found out when I got to the closing that I actually paid him $25,000 less than the mortgage he had on the land.

I asked Nick Garrison, who by then was living in Princeton, New Jersey, if he would design a new house for us in Georgia. He declined. "I've only built one house in my life, and that's your house for two up north," he explained. "I work for a big firm now, and I'd have to charge you far too much." But he agreed to do me a favour. "What I will do is come down and see the land you bought and the area that you'll be living in, and I'll sketch you a house. When that's done, I'll come back again and help you choose a local architect, but I won't be the architect of record." That's exactly what Nick did. He sketched the house in four drawings. They're now framed and hanging on a wall in the house down there. He came back down a second time to help us choose a local architect who, it turns out, was an American born in Montreal.

The house in Georgia is unique and quite marvellous. We call it "Porte Bonheur," the same name my mother gave to our family's beloved home in Murray Bay. From the outside, it looks like a traditional Quebec house with a Norman-style steep roof and dormer windows on the second floor. It's a style transplanted south like an architectural snowbird. You enter it by walking over a low bridge that connects the road with the house, which sits on stilts along the shore of Lake Clara, where twelve-foot-long alligators can sometimes be seen sunning themselves. The stilts are pylons of treated wood driven thirty feet into the ground and capped in cement. Although the house has a traditional look from the exterior, that's not the sense you get from it when you move inside. The house is designed on the principle that you should never build a house with more than one room in it, because you actually live in only one room. It's true that we have two bedrooms off the big main room and lofts above the bedrooms, but it's essentially one big space. The main room is twenty-five feet high from floor to ceiling, and we use it for everything – living room, dining room, kitchen, and laundry room all in one space. The purpose of the lofts is to sleep an infinite number of kids who love to clamber up the vertical ladders to their own world as soon as they arrive and don't need to go to the bathroom at night. The entire house is made of wood, no gypsum wallboard at all. The ceilings, walls, floors – everything is made of wood.

The house was finally finished in 2006 by which time I was only 82.

At the Ford Plantation development, many of the houses were built during the US real estate boom of a decade ago by people who no longer have the money to keep them up. There's one beautiful house that cost $3 million to build and then caught fire just as the owners were about to move in. They rebuilt it right away but then decided they weren't comfortable living in it. When they finally sold it, all they got was $850,000. It's going to be awhile until I can double or triple my money as I did with that house on Clarke Avenue. I realize that I now have a lovely house in Georgia that I couldn't sell for more than half of what I spent on it, but my kids love it, and I hope I'll be able to keep it. In any case, it's a bad idea to think you can ever make money out of private real estate. That's not why you buy a home to live in.

I particularly love visiting Georgia in the fall, which allows me to get back to Montreal and Lac Manitou in time for Christmas and the winter I still love. But by March, when winter has lost its charm and the gleam of fresh snow has turned into piles of grey frozen slush, I head south to the Georgia spring when the air is still fresh and before the onset of the sultry Southern summer.

Having become a new homeowner in my 80s, I think it may be time to slow down on the architecture front. More than forty years after building my first house, I've got no plans to build anything new, even if the dimensions are perfect.

6

"An Unobtrusive Jewel"

Building a Home for Alcan

A *Wall Street Journal* columnist once advised his readers never to buy the stock of a company whose C E O walks to work. The columnist's view was that any company run by a leader who had such a laid-back view of his work day couldn't be trusted to maximize what everybody these days loves to refer to by that awful term, shareholder value. If only that writer had found out about my commuting arrangements while at the helm of Alcan! The company would have instantly become a penny stock. For the almost thirty-five years that I worked for the company in Montreal, including ten years as C E O, I always walked to work from my home in Westmount to Alcan's downtown headquarters. It was the best thirty or forty minutes I spent every day, giving me time to contemplate big issues and small and do it on my own, without interruption. I knew that once I stepped into the office I would be constantly in meetings or on the phone with scarcely a moment on my own. The chance to be alone is the same reason I never minded long airplane trips.

As I made my way to work, at times I would think of nothing but the changing colours of the trees or the new blanket of snow on the slopes of Mount Royal. When my daughter Diane was in primary school, I would walk with her and drop her off at school en route. Even when I was assigned a chauffeur after being appointed C E O, I kept up the tradition. I would leave home with our two Labradors and walk briskly across Mount Royal Park, with the city's skyscrapers, the port, and the mighty St Lawrence River framed below in the distance. When we came off the mountain on Pine Avenue, my chauffeur would be there waiting to take the dogs home, and I would head down the hill to Alcan's offices at Place Ville Marie.

It was during those walks in the 1960s and 1970s that I saw the vast changes affecting Montreal as high-rise developments began to pop up everywhere. While I have never considered myself a blind opponent of progress, I was frankly appalled by some of the changes that were obliterating the history of my hometown and, in particular, the Sherbrooke Street that I had known and loved since I was a boy. In 1971, McGill University destroyed the Prince of Wales Terrace on the north side of Sherbrooke Street, one of the city's most historic buildings, in an act of vandalism unworthy of such a great institution. Inaugurated in 1860, it was named in honour of Albert Edward, Prince of Wales, who had travelled to Montreal to inaugurate the Victoria Bridge, named after his mother. The terrace consisted of nine townhouses with a classical Greek facade of Montreal limestone. The building was replaced by the insultingly bland and totally forgettable Samuel Bronfman Building, which houses McGill's management faculty. Then a couple of years later, the nearby Van Horne mansion, the onetime home of Sir William Van Horne, the legendary president of the Canadian Pacific Railway, also fell to the wrecker's ball, to be replaced by a nondescript office tower. This time, though, the public outrage sparked by the demolition helped launch Montreal's heritage preservation movement and led to the protection of other historic buildings from a similar fate.

Alcan itself had long had an association with architecture as a promoter of aluminum as a building product, whether in siding, windows, and doors or in more commercial applications like the aluminum panels used on the exterior curtain walls of skyscrapers. But, the company had never got around to building its own headquarters, preferring the flexibility and convenience of being a tenant. In the late 1950s, when Alcan was rapidly outgrowing its head office location in Montreal's Sun Life Building, the New York real estate developer William Zeckendorf came up with an audacious plan. For decades the centre of Montreal's downtown had been blighted by a giant seven-acre hole where the suburban railways and intercity passenger trains converged underground at Central Station. Zeckendorf's plan, drawn up in conjunction with the site's owner, Canadian National Railway, was to fill the hole with a giant commercial development that included a distinctive office tower to be built atop an underground shopping arcade, a revolutionary idea for the time.

Zeckendorf was a classic promoter who had developed a reputation for thinking big. He had assembled the land along New York's East River that became the site for the United Nations Headquarters building and later helped develop Century City in Los Angeles. An imposing man who always wore a black homburg, Zeckendorf came to see Nat Davis, Alcan's CEO, with a proposal. "Now, Mr Davis, we're going to build a great building in Montreal. We're going to fill that hole, and if Alcan becomes a major lease holder in the building, we'll use aluminum on the facade." Nat smiled at him sweetly and said, "Well, isn't it possible that you'd use aluminum anyway?" Zeckendorf responded, "Mr Davis, you know how these things go. We've got to find some big tenants." Then he proposed that Alcan invest directly in the project. Nat, attempting to sound interested, said, "What are you thinking of, five million dollars?" Zeckendorf looked at him and in his booming voice responded, "Nat, for five million all you get is a white chip." This was one poker game that Nat decided was not for him, but, nevertheless, Alcan ended up signing a twenty-year lease for eight floors of what was to become Place Ville Marie, for a time the largest office building in the Commonwealth. When Alcan moved into the complex at its opening in 1963, Mr Powell, who headed Alcan's principal subsidiary, Aluminum Co. of Canada, was really annoyed to discover that the main tower had been named for the Royal Bank of Canada while Alcan's presence was virtually ignored. He figured that securing our lease was just as important to the project, if not more so, as the Royal Bank's decision to move its headquarters up the hill from St James Street.

Place Ville Marie proved to be a great looking building, clad in aluminum even though Alcan never became an investor, and it looks as good today as it did half a century ago. The Chinese-American architect I.M. Pei and his colleague Henry Cobb did a great job with the design. Talk about good architecture. The dimensions of that building are extraordinary. The cruciform main tower standing in the middle of a large plaza meant there were tons of corner offices and lots of outdoor space. Zeckendorf had tremendous vision. He hired good architects and didn't scrimp on materials. For me, the test of good architecture is if every time you set foot in a building, it feels like the first time. And, that's the sense I still get the moment I walk into the lobby of Place Ville Marie.

For Zeckendorf, as for many visionary developers, his tremendous foresight and guts didn't translate into financial success. He went bankrupt a couple of times, and Place Ville Marie was always a sketchy financial proposition for him. I remember *Time* magazine once asking Zeckendorf if it was true that he was paying eighteen per cent for money to finance his ventures. Zeckendorf retorted, "I won't answer the question, but I'll tell you this, I'd rather be alive at eighteen per cent than dead at five per cent."

The future of Alcan's head office became one of the first questions I had to deal with when I took over as C E O in the middle of 1979. When we had moved into Place Ville Marie in 1963, Alcan signed a twenty-year lease at a base rent of $5 per square foot. By 1979, with just over three years to run on the lease, the landlord was warning me that the new rent would be $24 per square foot, or almost five times the amount we'd been paying. There was another issue as well. The 1976 election of the Parti Québécois government of René Lévesque had sparked a massive exodus of head offices like Sun Life down highway 401 to Toronto. And with the referendum on separation expected in the spring of 1980, things were only getting worse. Skittish employees were constantly coming into my office and asking me, "Are we going or are we staying?" I would respond calmly, "Of course we're staying. This is just one of many different governments that we'll have in Quebec. Our roots are very deep in this province, and there's no question that we're stay-ing." Yet I could sense those employees were leaving my office unconvinced and thinking to themselves, "Well, what else can he say? He has to say we're staying." I felt that the only way I could convince them that Alcan was committed to remaining in Quebec was to build our own head office in Montreal. It was an idea that had been percolating in my brain for some time, but now I felt the time had come to act. It was the summer of 1979.

The following day I got together with Hugh Norsworthy, one of the thirteen Harvard M B A graduates who, with me, had joined Alcan in July of 1949. I told him that Alcan needed to build its own head office in downtown Montreal. I also thought that it should serve as a catalyst for the further protection and restoration of the glory of Sherbrooke Street, which had been maimed over the years by out-of-control demolition. "I have an idea we should try and start with the Atholstan House on the corner of Sherbrooke and Stanley," I told him.

Built in 1895 for Sir Hugh Graham, who later became Lord Atholstan, founder of *The Montreal Star* newspaper, the house was an imposing four-storey stone mansion with classical styling that wouldn't have been out of place on New York's Fifth Avenue. It had subsequently been owned by the Jesuit religious order before being bought by the Shah of Iran as part of a network of Iran Houses, in London, Paris, New York, and Los Angeles, set up to showcase the glory and power of his kingdom. With opposition to the Shah's regime growing, there was also suspicion that his entou-rage might be interested in using the house as a safe harbour if he ever had to leave Iran in a hurry and flee to the West. There was even a secret exit built into the house, which had been dubbed Maison de l'Iran. By 1979, after a few half-hearted attempts at ren-ovations, the building had been virtually abandoned, the Shah had fled his country, and the new Islamic government, led by Ayatollah Khomeini, didn't seem much interested in owning a 13,000 square foot mansion in downtown Montreal. A classified ad had actually appeared in *The Montreal Star* offering a "large prestigious prop-erty" that could be used as "a consulate, cultural and research centre, offices, boutiques." Yet despite its forlorn look, it seemed to me that a refurbished Atholstan House could be transformed into the perfect home for the executive group that ran Alcan worldwide.

That morning in August of 1979, I called Derek Drummond, head of the School of Architecture at McGill and scion of an old Montreal family, and asked him if he had an hour to come over and talk with us. I immediately asked Derek whom I should use as an architect, and he started with Arthur Erickson and went down the list of the top names in Canada. But after half an hour of mulling over the list, nothing had clicked. Then, almost off-handedly, Derek made another suggestion, "Maybe we should throw in Ray Affleck's name. He's the one we call Mr Sherbrooke Street. He loves Sherbrooke Street." And I responded, "That's my man!" Ray Affleck, a founder of the Arcop architecture practice, was already an accomplished architect credited with such important buildings as the Place des Arts cultural complex and the Place Bonaventure trade and convention center in Montreal as well as the National Arts Centre in Ottawa.

I arranged to meet Ray and began going through the process of figuring out what I was going to say to this man, knowing that what I would say at the beginning was going to determine what the end would look like. It took me a few days, but I finally hit on a phrase. I started our first meeting by saying, "Ray, you know Alcan is a big company by Canadian standards, and most big companies like to build skyscrapers, but we don't want a skyscraper. Our purpose is to make it very clear to the people working for Alcan that we're staying in Montreal. Therefore, we want something that looks like a home. We don't want to make a massive statement of any kind. In fact, what I'd like you to build for Alcan is an unobtrusive jewel." And, that's what we got in the end. That phrase, an unobtrusive jewel, is what's on a plaque in the atrium at Maison Alcan. Rather than assemble a group of properties with the aim of tearing them down to build a massive new structure, my goal was to purchase an "ensemble" of older buildings, refurbish, restore, and reuse them, tying them together into an understated new international home for Alcan.

Affleck thought this was a fine idea, but he knew it wouldn't be enough simply to get our hands on the Atholstan mansion, which could house a handful of Alcan executives and their staff, a total of about fifty people, but nowhere near the hundreds working at Place Ville Marie. "If you get Atholstan House, that's only the beginning. You're going to need a lot more space than that." I agreed, not realizing that Alcan would end up buying half a dozen separate properties covering much of a block of downtown Montreal. "Okay, but anything we want we'd better buy before May 1980, because after the referendum property prices are going to start going up again."

Thus began one of the most fascinating experiences in my business career, during which I remained the C E O of Canada's most prominent multinational while at the same time took on the cloak-and-dagger role of a property developer quietly accumulating real estate without anybody catching on. To assemble the properties, I turned to an old acquaintance, Leslie Gault, who probably didn't have a real estate license but had been buying smaller properties for himself around Montreal for a while. It may have not been strictly kosher, but I knew we had to act with the utmost discretion. Leslie was a few years older than I was, a country gentleman type who had married a well-to-do English woman. I figured he wouldn't raise suspicion. He was my "beard."

Montreal's economy at the time was in a state of limbo. Many big companies had left for Toronto, and the ones that remained were not investing, but waiting for the outcome of the referendum expected the following spring. Every second property was for sale and at very good prices. Construction of a massive new Holiday Inn, later to become a Sheraton hotel, on nearby Dorchester Boulevard had been halted for years, an abandoned concrete hulk that was a potent symbol of the uncertainty that had overtaken the city's economy. But I knew that once the referendum had passed, presuming that the separatists lost, prices were likely to shoot up, and my unobtrusive jewel would soon be as pricey as the Hope diamond. It was essential to move quickly and under the radar. Without fanfare, Alcan set up a numbered company with the objective "to acquire the appropriate properties, land and buildings to create new distinct head office premises for Alcan Group headquarters." Internally, we began to refer to the venture as "Project X."

Leslie got to work and found it surprisingly easy to get hold of the Maison de l'Iran, even though there were three mortgages on the property, one of which was in default, and a contractor had registered a lien on the house for unpaid renovation work. But even if the Iranians were willing sellers, I still had visions of building our new headquarters on the site and in ten or fifteen years' time looking out the window one day and seeing hundreds of angry students with placards accusing Alcan of stealing the building from the people of Iran in their moment of trial. I insisted that the deed of sale be signed by a senior official in the Khomeini government, and so it was a short time later that Iran's new Minister of National Guidance for Information and Publicity authorized the sale of Maison de l'Iran to our numbered company.

Just behind Atholstan House was an empty lot that belonged to the fellow who owned LaSalle College, a private vocational school. He was pleased to find a buyer for the property and agreed to let it go for $450,000. When I was a student, it had been the site of some brothels, but now it was just a parking lot. Then Leslie bought the lovely townhouse next to Atholstan House on Sherbrooke Street; it had a grey stone facade and had been built in 1894 for an old French Canadian family, the Béiques. We also bought a bit of the lane behind the house.

Things were going well. Then Ray Affleck told me we'd have to try to acquire the Berkeley Hotel if there was going to be enough space. The Berkeley was a ten-storey, brick-faced building built in the 1920s as bachelor apartments for young single men. The rooms had no kitchens. The venture had failed, and the building had been converted into a hotel with a lobby bar that became very popular with students from nearby McGill University. But the Berkeley had since fallen on hard times and closed. Here, Leslie ran into a real problem. There was a watchman sitting in the hotel lobby but no other sign of life. As the months passed, Leslie tried repeatedly to discover the owner's identity but had no success. He couldn't get past a law office to find out who the beneficial owner was. Then in early 1980 Leslie, in desperation, went once again to the law office. The lawyer told him, "Look, quit bugging me. All I can tell you is that the owner is European," adding ominously that his mysterious client was having a development study conducted on what could be done with the Berkeley Hotel and was not going to make a decision on selling until the study had been completed.

I figured we had to act quickly. I told Leslie to buy the house on the western side of the hotel along Sherbrooke Street. We already had the Atholstan and Béique houses on the eastern side of the hotel, and if we could get the Holland House to the west, we'd have our mystery guy surrounded, and his development study would never end up going anywhere. Leslie called me back a couple of hours later with some bad news, "We're too late. The Holland house, the lane behind it, and two small commercial buildings on Drummond Street have just been sold for $500,000." (That's the price of a modest home in a nice Montreal suburb these days.) I told Les, "Call him back and offer him $800,000." Les was incredulous. I said "Yes, I'll give him $800,000 but only if he'll sell right away." He called me back an hour later and said, "You've got it. The owner is delighted. He's made a nice profit and he's very happy."

Things were falling into place like those little tokens in a Monopoly game. We had purchased several properties and had the Berkeley Hotel surrounded. Yet we still couldn't find out who owned the old hotel. So, on 10 February 1980, with the May referendum lurking around the corner, I decided to do something desperate. Alcan had just hired a new head of security who had come from the Canadian Armed Forces and had served for a time as a security officer for N A T O. I said to him, "Paul, I've got to find out who owns the Berkeley Hotel. All I know is that he's European, possibly Italian." Twenty minutes later Paul called me back and said, "If you go over to the Sonesta Hotel on the corner of Peel and Sherbrooke, in Room 1141 you'll find an Italian gentleman who checked in yesterday at 4 p.m. He owns the Berkeley Hotel." Until this day, I don't know where Paul got that crucial piece of intelligence. I never asked.

I immediately called Leslie Gault. "Get yourself over to the Sonesta Hotel and look up an Italian gentleman in Room 1141. And tell him most of the truth. Tell him that you've dabbled in real estate and that you now own and control the Atholstan House, the Béique House, and the Holland House, and offer him $2 million for the Berkeley Hotel provided he'll give you an answer in one hour." Les said, "Are you serious?" I responded, "Damned right, I'm serious." Les called me back about an hour later and reported, "Charming gentleman. I offered him the $2 million if he'd take it in an hour. He walked around the room twice, smiled at me, put out his hand, and said you've got a deal." The deal finally closed on 16 May, four days before the Quebec referendum. At that point, including the acquisition cost for the Berkeley Hotel, we had paid just under $5 million for everything – the Atholstan House, the land and the lane behind, the Béique House, the Berkeley Hotel, the Holland House and the property adjacent to it on Drummond Street. Less than $5 million for a prime site on Canada's grandest street. That tells you what real estate values were before the referendum.

While we managed to keep a cone of silence over the project, my idea of building a new headquarters in Quebec when the threat of political separation hung heavily in the air was not embraced with enthusiasm by everybody at Alcan. As for the board, I'm still not sure how I got away with it. Denys Simmons, Alcan's treasurer, wrote a handwritten two-page memo pleading with me to reconsider. "Is it wise to commit prior to the referendum?" he wrote, warning that, "to do so may have political significance." He worried that going ahead with Project X would appear to be giving tacit approval to Quebec's onerous personal income tax rates and that the high-profile location of the complex on Sherbrooke Street could make Alcan, "vulnerable to demonstrations, picketing, and vandalism by extremists in the labour force." Rather than take the risk he argued, "Could we not extend our Place Ville Marie lease to allow more time?" Even after the project got its final go-ahead, John Hale, executive vice president of finance, wrote to me confidentially warning that the new headquarters represented, "a very firm commitment for Alcan's head office to stay in Quebec" and would weaken Alcan's bargaining position with the provincial government when it came to problems like tax, language, and education. A few executives even objected to the name of the complex, Maison Alcan, with one protesting that the name had the ring of, "a high-class restaurant or a couturier." In the end, we decided that, while the complex would be called Maison Alcan, the company's official letterhead address would be simply 1188 Sherbrooke Street West.

I was well aware of the political risks but still convinced I was on the right track. In seeking approval from the Alcan Executive Committee for Project X, it was made clear that if Alcan's head office were to leave Montreal at some time in the future, "the problem of vacated premises would be minor compared to the human and political problems. Certainly, the reality of our hydropower and smelter investments in the Saguenay dictate that Alcan will always have a major headquarters for Quebec operations in this city. Hence, in the unlikely event of world headquarters moving away, the proposed facilities could be readily adapted and occupied by the management and staff that remain to manage Quebec operations." In the end, thankfully, we never had to deal with that eventuality.

With the properties assembled, we continued to push forward. My initial vision was to move Alcan's international headquarters to the new complex, which would include the three old houses we had purchased as well as the Berkeley Hotel. These four buildings on Sherbrooke would be linked at the back by a four-storey atrium that would also provide access to a new seven-storey office structure that we decided to call the Davis Building, in honour of the family of our founding CEO. Staff from Alcan's main Canadian subsidiaries would stay behind at Place Ville Marie. The atrium would also house boutiques and provide space for cultural events like art exhibits and concerts.

On 20 May 1980, Quebecers soundly rejected the separatist option in the much-anticipated referendum by a three-to-two margin. Just over a week later, on 29 May, Alcan issued a news release announcing plans for a new headquarters building on Sherbrooke Street in downtown Montreal, noting that the property assembly had only been completed two weeks earlier, on 16 May. In the news release, I was quoted as saying, "We have spent more than six months assembling property so we could develop a project which we believe will preserve and enhance a section of downtown Montreal. We expect our plans to meet the approval of the people of Montreal."

Project X had been a complete success. Not a word about it had leaked in advance, and the press and public reaction was enthusiastic to say the least. Even before construction began, Maison Alcan was a hit with employees, architectural mavens, and the general public. "Hats off to Alcan," wrote the Montreal *Gazette* in an editorial. "Its choice of this site recalls the sophistication of some of the large European firms which make their homes in tasteful historic structures." I even got a highly congratulatory letter from Denis Vaugeois, the Quebec Cultural Affairs Minister and outspoken nationalist, who expressed his admiration of Alcan for its respect for Quebec's architectural heritage.

A short time later, Ray Affleck rented a helicopter and positioned it above all the properties that we had purchased. Looking down, he could see the Salvation Army Citadel, as its church was known, on Drummond Street at the back of our site. On the north side of the Citadel, the Salvation Army had built some wooden shacks (to use as offices) that were an eyesore and even obscured the stained glass windows of the church. Ray said to me, "David, why don't we tell the Salvation Army that if they'll sell us the Citadel and the land under those shacks, we'll keep the Citadel and get rid of those lean-tos and expose their lovely stained glass windows. We'll also build them an office building on Stanley Street in the same style as the Davis Building. We'll charge them a Chevrolet price for a Cadillac building." After some tough negotiations, we finally got a deal, which included completing the ensemble with a pleasantly landscaped public walkway linking Stanley and Drummond Streets between the Davis building and the Citadel. With the addition of the Salvation Army component and an expanded Davis

Building, by the time ground was broken the next spring, the size of the project had grown to 396,000 square feet and the cost was estimated at $40 million. And, despite the complexities of dealing with the integration of a series of old and new structures, the project was completed within that estimate. To this day there are people, some whom I know and some whose names are unknown to me, who tell me how much they appreciate the few moments of détente they experience as they walk through the passage between the Citadel and the Davis building. The birds like it too.

Of course, in any venture of this scale, there is always a holdout. We quickly realized that Walter Klinkhoff, owner of one of Canada's best known art galleries, was not interested in selling his property, a greystone townhouse just west of Holland House. "It was not a question of money," Walter insisted in a newspaper interview at the time. "I've got something I've always wanted, and it's the best location in the city." His gallery had opened in 1955, and he was initially a tenant until he managed to buy the townhouse from the real estate speculator who wanted to demolish the building. "We're so happy to own the place after years of bad experiences as tenants that we just couldn't imagine selling," he said. There was more. Walter, who was an acquaintance of mine and a sometime tennis partner, engaged in a long correspondence with the supremely patient Hugh Norsworthy in which he complained about the disruption to his gallery business, the limits on his parking, and even his hatred of Muzak, all of which he blamed on the Alcan project. Discussing the fact that the back wall of his building would have access to the Maison Alcan atrium, Walter noted, "I detest piped-in music whether in planes, elevators, restaurants or shopping malls. I compare it to force-feeding and I am immediately possessed by the irresistible urge to escape." He said that since the gallery would probably have to keep its windows open for ventilation, if music were to be piped into the atrium, "it could be borne in mind that my particular preference is Mozart, Beethoven and the classical opera repertoire." In the end, we agreed to build several underground parking spaces for Klinkhoff to compensate him for the loss of his laneway and to lease the upper floors of the gallery building from him. But otherwise we left him alone, with his property intact, as long as he gave Alcan a right of first refusal if he ever chose to sell. Walter has since passed away but his sons still run the gallery, which continues to boast the best location in the city.

The design for Maison Alcan came together quite quickly and construction was completed by July of 1983, three years after the original announcement. In addition to Ray Affleck, I used an old Westmount interior decorating firm, called Iron Cat, to help locate furniture, antiques, and artworks that would be appropriate for the older parts of the complex, particularly Atholstan House, where the executive offices were to be located. I put the owner of Iron Cat together with a young Montreal architect named Julia Gersovitz who had studied historic preservation at Columbia and helped restore Atholstan House and the other existing buildings to their original glory. To add to the authenticity, the McCord Museum kindly lent me Lord Atholstan's own desk for my office. To top off the accolades from the community at large, Maison Alcan was awarded a Prix d'Excellence from Quebec's Order of Architects in 1984. Soon after the headquarters staff moved into Maison Alcan, the world was hit with a serious recession and Alcan wasn't spared, forcing a downsizing of headquarters staff through early retirements and layoffs. That freed up space in the new headquarters for employees of the Canadian smelting and fabricating arm, so in the end they too made the move from Place Ville Marie to Sherbrooke Street, bringing everybody under the same roof.

Thirty years later, I still feel like a proud father every time I enter Maison Alcan, which is just down the street from my current office. But, I admit to a twinge of regret that Alcan's current owners have closed the building off from the public. The atrium, where once there were lunchtime concerts and art exhibitions, is strangely silent, and the shaded walkway that links Stanley and Drummond Streets alongside the old Salvation Army Citadel is now locked shut at night with a large steel gate. Likewise, the once-animated gallery of shops has been closed. Maison Alcan may still be a jewel but one whose sparkle is no longer shared with the community at large.

With the completion of Maison Alcan, the company's involvement with architecture didn't end. One day in the 1980s, I was sitting in my office at Atholstan House and in walked Phyllis Lambert, the daughter of Samuel Bronfman, who had made her name as an architect, philanthropist, and astute businesswoman. "You know I have a pretty good collection of architectural drawings, and I've decided to build a home to put them in," she told me. "It's going to cost me $76 million to build. I'm putting in $70 million. Would you help me raise $6 million?" I agreed that Alcan would play its part.

When I was asked by the Alcan board to explain, I responded, "How many of you guys have ever been in that situation? A nice lady walks in and says I'm going to do something that's great for Montreal, I'm going to pay $70 million and asks me to help her raise $6 million." The board wondered what I had in mind, and I responded, "I think Alcan should give her $2 million." To which they replied, "We've never given $2 million to anything!" I explained that this would be a unique attribute for Montreal. I won the argument and Alcan ended up giving $2 million toward the Canadian Centre for Architecture. Phyllis gave me two naming opportunities, one for a study centre that was to bring leading architects from all over the world to Montreal for a period of time with their families, and the other for a theatre. I chose the study centre because any city that hosts the best architectural minds over a period of time should end up reflecting that influence.

Working with Phyllis required a certain degree of self-confidence. She's one smart woman, but she has a real capacity to put you down, and if you let it get to you it must be terrible. Not only does she not suffer fools, she doesn't suffer many people. But, she's a great person, and what she does is so extraordinary that people who work for her become captivated by her vision and learn how to stand the heat in the kitchen.

By choosing to build the Canadian Centre for Architecture where she did, in the long-abandoned Shaughnessy House mansion situated in a deserted bit of downtown Montreal near the entrance of an expressway, she really did her part in trying to kick-start urban regeneration. She's also been trying steadfastly to improve the rest of that neighbourhood, and in particular the terrible part of Sainte-Catherine between Atwater and Guy near the old Forum where her nephew, Stephen Bronfman, Charles's son, is active in condo development.

Despite Phyllis's efforts and the improvements on Sherbooke Street that have come following the construction of Maison Alcan, I remain disappointed that it hasn't spurred the kind of interest in quality architecture that I would have hoped for. It's not just an issue in Montreal. It reflects complacency about good design that is evident across Canada. I'll give you two current examples in Montreal. One is the new McGill University Health Centre (MUHC), a massive new project in the city's west end on the site of the Glen Yard, a former Canadian Pacific rail yard. When I became chairman of the MUHC board in 2000, I believed the Glen Yard project would be finished by 2009, and I innocently thought that the hospital itself was going to be able to build it. I lined up Moshe Safdie as the architect. Because of the new hospital's location on a cliff overlooking the major transportation routes entering Montreal and the St Lawrence River beyond, I figured that the Glen Yard Site had the potential to be associated with Montreal the way the Sydney Opera House is associated with Sydney, Australia. With his Montreal roots and his international achievements over the decades, beginning with Habitat at Expo 67 just after graduating from McGill, I thought Safdie would be the ideal person to create such a statement.

In the end, it was just too imaginative an approach for the Quebec government. Little did I know that the Quebec government, the major funder of the healthcare system, would never let the MUHC build the hospital and that the project would be delayed by a decade. I was clearly told by Quebec's finance minister that the government would decide everything. Safdie withdrew his name. At Quebec's behest, the McGill project is being built by a private-public partnership with the architecture simply treated as an afterthought. The consortium will deliver a hospital that I'm certain is going to be very good on the inside, but I'm afraid the outside will look like a modern Bordeaux jail. Unfortunately, it's the outside that will be seen by every visitor to Montreal driving in from the airport for the rest of time, whereas with a little bit of effort it could have been designed to make a lasting impression. I feel the same sense of missed opportunity with the recent opening of the Montreal Symphony Orchestra's concert hall. After years of dreaming of a custom-built home for classical music, it finally became a reality. The inside is great, with excellent acoustics, but the outside looks like a warehouse squished into a corner of the Place des Arts cultural complex. It would have probably been a bit more expensive to build a better quality hall, but the impact on the city would have been all that much more lasting and, dare I say, inspiring.

I, for one, believe that good architecture pays for itself many times over the generations.

7

"On Hands and Knees"

Developing Ties with Japan and China

When I set foot in Japan for the first time in 1957, it was just a dozen years after the devastation of the Second World War, and the country's economy was still in development. Tokyo was dusty, dirty, and noisy. The streets were bustling and jammed with two-wheeled and three-wheeled motorcycles carrying tons of steel on flat tires. It was helter-skelter.

Yet it was evident even in those days that this was a very special place, a civilization with a storied history and culture, and an economy with fabulous potential. My first night in Japan, after the long flight across the Pacific on a Canadian Pacific Airlines DC-4, I had been invited to dinner by the last remaining member of the Tokugawa family, the dynasty that had run Japan between 1603 and 1868. Prince Iemasa Tokugawa had been named Japan's ambassador to Canada in 1929 when the two countries exchanged diplomatic representatives for the first time. As an indication of the importance Canada's political leaders placed on Japan, Tokyo was only the third place outside the Commonwealth where Canada set up its own embassy after cutting its diplomatic apron strings with Britain in the 1920s. The other two were Washington and Paris. As for the Japanese, they had decided to dispatch the prince as far away from Japan as possible so that there would be no temptation for him to get into politics.

While in Ottawa, the prince used to come frequently to Montreal for visits and to stay at the Place Viger Hotel, the Chateau-style railway hotel in Old Montreal that has long since lost its original vocation. At the time, my mother was a well-known hostess, and, during his sojourns in Montreal, the prince became a frequent dinner guest at our home. During the course of one of those visits, Prince Tokugawa became enamoured of a married lady who was also a friend of my mother. Over the following few years, Fern would often receive a phone call from the Japanese embassy in Ottawa asking her to arrange a dinner party on the following Saturday night and to include the prince's lady friend in the guest list. It was the way things were done at the time. The prince clearly appreciated my mother's help in arranging these rendezvous.

Years later, when my mother heard that the first stop on my worldwide tour would be Tokyo, she said to me, "I know someone there who owes me a favour, and I'm going to write to him and tell him that you're coming." When I arrived in Tokyo, an invitation to dinner with Prince Tokugawa was waiting for me at my hotel. As it turned out, I was deathly ill and hardly in the mood for a night on the town. I had been given something like twenty-nine inoculations before the trip and they had all erupted in me during the flight. I knew I had to go to this dinner, which was to be held in a classical geisha house in Akasaka in central Tokyo. I entered what was a large room for Japan, with one small table in the middle set for eight people. The prince sat me on his left, and there was one empty spot, which he explained to me would be filled by a Mr Komatsu, who had been invited to the dinner because he had attended Monmouth College in Illinois with my father-in-law Rip Powell many decades earlier. Only the Japanese would go to the trouble to do such extensive research simply to find an ideal guest for a dinner meeting with a perfect stranger arriving from another continent.

We began dinner, and finally Komatsu arrived. The little screen doorway in the corner of the big room slid open. In came Komatsu on his hands and knees. At which point, the five other Japanese gentlemen who had been sitting at the table, everybody except the prince, pushed away from the table and also fell on their hands and knees. They started crawling toward Komatsu who was coming towards them from the far corner. When they met, still on their hands and knees, the six men in business suits and ties started exchanging business cards, their meishi. By that time, my eyes were bulging. I had never seen anything like it. Then Komatsu looked up and said in excellent English, "Mr Culver, what do you think of our Japanese habits?" At which point, sitting to my right, Prince Tokugawa said, "Komatsu, can you not speak Japanese?" The prince was clearly irritated to hear English being spoken during this key moment in any Japanese business encounter. It was a clear breach of etiquette as he saw it. I said to myself that this was a complex society that would take me a long time to understand. Over the course of the next five decades I visited Japan on at least fifty occasions, and I still feel I have not have reached a full comprehension of the place and its people.

To understand Japan, it's useful to think of it not as a nation, like Canada or the United States, but as a tribe with very strong tribal customs. Because it's so natural for Japan to maintain its rigid and prescribed customs, there is always a great danger of isolationism, which has been so damaging to the country in the past. Before that first visit to Tokyo in 1957, I read a *Time Magazine* article by a correspondent who decided as part of his research into Japanese society to look into the legendary political power of the farm lobby. His first stop was to contact an old farmer. The reporter asked the farmer for his impression of General Douglas MacArthur, Supreme Commander of Allied Powers during the occupation of Japan in the aftermath of the Second World War. The farmer's answer was this, "The Emperor could not have chosen a better man." Considering the fact that for most of us in the West, Emperor Hirohito had been humiliated by the US occupation, it was an amazing statement. But for this elderly farmer, the Emperor remained a deity, and everything, including the American occupation of Japan, was somehow still his handiwork. It also illustrates the inherent isolationism of Japan, a phenomenon I thought was dangerous for the world's second largest economy. I became convinced that I would try to do my part to encourage

Japan to reject that isolationism and increase its engagement with the world, not just for its own sake but also for the sake of us all.

From its earliest days, Alcan had been active in Japan. With no bauxite and no supply of cheap electric power, Japan was an early importer of the metal. In fact, the first export shipment from Alcan's pioneering smelter in Shawinigan, Quebec in 1901 was a sale of 67,000 pounds of ingot sent to Yokohama, Japan. Alcoa continued to develop close relations with Japan and was fortunate to have talented managers like Elmer MacDowell, my future boss in international sales, on hand to develop the business. MacDowell barely escaped the Yokohama earthquake of 1923, having by chance travelled to Tokyo that day to look for a telegram from headquarters. When he returned to Yokohama, the residence where he had been staying was no more, and the dozen men with whom he had eaten breakfast the day before had been killed. A colleague at Alcoa, Jack King, also survived, but his wife and daughter were killed by the catastrophe.

Shortly after its spinoff as a separate company in 1928, Alcan signed a partnership agreement with the Sumitomo Group to establish an aluminum sheet and foil operation. We lost contact with the firm during the war, but the minute the war ended we were back in business again. It all went well until 1953 when the Japanese government invited us to take a fifty per cent interest in Nippon Light Metal, which operated an aluminum smelter. This caused a profound crisis of loyalty for Alcan. The problem was that Nippon Light Metal was part of the Furukawa Group, a rival to Sumitomo. A raging debate took place within Alcan as to whether this offer of a fifty per cent interest in Nippon Light Metal should be accepted or not. The old Japan hands at Alcan thought it was a bad idea. They strongly believed that if you had an understanding with the Sumitomo Group, you didn't sign an understanding with another group. In other words, you shouldn't have two wives. But, Nippon was a much bigger venture than the foil company, and the price was very cheap. In the end, North American pragmatism won over Japanese tradition, and we decided to take up the offer

and buy into the smelter. Thereafter followed many awkward
years for Alcan in Japan, particularly among the expatriate staff
who had trouble dividing their loyalty. There was a noticeable lack
of trust between those in Alcan working with Nippon Light Metal
and those working with Sumitomo.

The president of Sumitomo Light Metal, Alcan's biggest customer in Japan, was Tanaka-san, whom I met during my first trip
to Japan in 1957. On my second day in the country, he took me on
a personal tour of Kyoto and then brought me to a geisha house for
dinner. We were a small group of four and Mr Tanaka decided to
test out his pretty basic command of English on me. As we began
to sip our cups of sake, Mr Tanaka toasted the occasion and said,
"So sorry Mrs Culver not with you." As the evening wore on and
the sake kept on flowing, Mr Tanaka lifted his cup again and said,
"So happy Mrs Culver not with you." He had a great sense of
humour; a man with a trustful and slightly wicked face.

A couple of years later, Mr Tanaka travelled to Montreal with
his wife and daughter, Teruko, who must have been only eighteen
or nineteen at the time and served as interpreter for her father.
Recognizing Sumitomo's standing as a leading customer, Alcan's
C E O, Nathanael Davis, hosted a dinner party for the Tanakas at
the Mount Royal Club. Nat was a terribly nice man but a bit shy
and retiring, so it was sometimes difficult for him to get the conversation going with small talk. All this led to some awkward
moments with his Japanese guests. Then Teruko piped up and
said, "Mr Davis, my father thinks that he's an important man
because he's president of Sumitomo Light Metal Industries, but,
actually, he's an important man because he's the second vice president of the Japan Lawn Tennis Association." That got everybody
laughing and broke the ice. After that, Teruko became my closest
friend in Japan. Every time I went to Japan I would visit her and
her husband, a Japanese lawyer who also happened to be a member of the English Bar, an unusual combination. That friendship
outlasted her father's career at Sumitomo and continues to this
day. Thanks to Teruko, over the years I learned more about

Japanese society than I could ever have done from my cordial but rather formal relations with business colleagues.

I've made as many as fifty trips to Japan over the past five decades, with visits sometimes twice a year, although never for more than four or five days at a time. Tokyo has figured in almost every trip but also Osaka, Kobe, and occasionally Sapporo. You have to be patient in developing business in Japan, to be slow, and deliberate. You have to develop trust and be transparent. It's true the Japanese love intrigue, but I'm not smart enough to play games. Japan doesn't exist to make money for foreign companies. Because they're so afraid of the word "no," the Japanese have traditionally been terrible sellers. A good salesman has to be immune to the repeated rejections he must endure before a buyer says yes. Yet that same fear of rejection is also why the Japanese end up being good buyers. That's one reason they developed the trading company system. While its initial purpose was to limit the corrupting influence of foreigners on Japanese society by restraining the number of businessmen exposed to the outside, the system also ended up limiting to a small group of trading companies those who would be forced to live with the world of "no." They could live abroad, becoming partly foreign and getting used to it.

I retain great respect for the Japanese ability to work together as a team in business. They take a long time to make up their minds to do something, but once they decide that they're going to do it, they act very quickly. They will develop a new product in a research lab, and once they decide it's ready to sell, they tend to get it on the market much faster than we do. They often will pick up the equipment that they've used in the lab for the development phase and simply cart it over, as is, to the manufacturing plant nearby, set it down, and put it into production. They're very efficient and have some of the best assembly-line workers that you could possibly want.

Despite my frequent visits, I never learned the Japanese language, in part because I had a man representing the Alcan sales organization in Japan who went all the way the other way.

Jack Boetschi already spoke at least five languages when he was first posted to Japan, and then he picked up Japanese in the most complete and impressive way. I'm talking not just about mastering the language to order a meal in a restaurant or conduct a business meeting but to the extent of becoming an expert in Japanese calligraphy, martial arts, and traditional long songs. Jack would go to a geisha party along with his Japanese colleagues and dress up as a samurai warrior. Then he would get up and sing these long songs, used in Kabuki theatre, which the Japanese themselves often find too difficult to sing. But there are limits to "going native," especially in Japan. Once when Jack was performing at one of these parties, the Japanese man beside me said, "Mr Culver, what do you think the people of Scotland would think if I were to turn up in a kilt and begin singing Scottish songs better than they could?" In other words, he thought that this Westerner had gone too far.

During my early visits to Japan, I would sometimes go to geisha parties nightly. In those early years, when a man was named president of a Japanese company, one of the first things he would do was decide what geisha house he was going to use for entertaining. It was not really his choice. It was the decision of the mama-san, the lady in charge of the geisha house, to figure out which executives she would accept as patrons. There was a good reason for this. So many of a company's innermost secrets were discussed at geisha parties that the mama-san would not want information overheard by the geishas at these parties to be shared with the company's competitors. Once a geisha house had been selected, it was an exclusive arrangement and you were always invited to the same geisha house by the same company. The company president would usually sponsor his own geisha. These women would be highly indebted by the time they completed their apprenticeships, owing the mama-san plenty of money for their kimonos, their training in music and dance, and everything else that is required to become an accomplished practitioner of the art. In these cases, the wealthy corporate patron would help pay off the debts of his favourite geisha as part of the arrangement.

This businessman and patron would probably attend his preferred geisha house two or three nights a week and be treated to excellent food and copious amounts of alcohol. There used to be a fifty per cent tax on everything you consumed if you stayed later than 9:30 p.m., which meant it was pretty well guaranteed you'd be ushered out of the place by that time. To continue the night's entertainment, you would then be taken directly to a Western-style bar for brandy and scotch. In the early days, the geishas, who usually spoke only Japanese, had trouble figuring out how to entertain their foreign guests. Their solution was to dream up a lot of silly games. I remember one geisha would take a bowl full of dried peas and an empty bowl and have a race with you to see who could move the dried peas with chopsticks faster from one bowl to the other. All this simply to pass the time until 9:30.

But as the years went on, geisha houses became too expensive as a form of corporate entertainment, and they were used less and less. As a result, there are fewer and fewer geisha houses and fewer girls going into the business. It's a very onerous life, described so beautifully in the book *Memoirs of a Geisha*, to which fewer young Japanese women are willing to commit.

As Japan's economy soared in the 1970s and Canadians began to take notice, Alcan was in the privileged position of having a long and successful history with Japanese business. It was a rare opportunity and one that placed a special responsibility on the company to help nurture the Canada-Japan relationship. As president of the Aluminum Co. of Canada, I was delighted to be asked by Jean Chrétien, then the federal minister of Industry, Trade and Commerce, to become the Canadian cochairman of the Canada Japan Business Committee when it was set up in 1976. Another key reason why I was pleased to become involved in the group was that my Japanese cochairman was Hisao Makita, chairman of the second largest steel company in Japan, Nippon Kokan. Mr Makita was a man who in many ways reminded me of my father. The Japanese don't respect youth particularly, so when I first met Mr Makita in his office in Tokyo, he was very kind to me, and not once did he show disappointment that he thought I was a bit of a kid to be doing this. I was about fifty, a real youngster, while Mr Makita must have been in his late sixties. We worked together on this business group for the next eleven years.

Mr Makita clearly felt the same way about the importance of our personal relationship to the success of the committee. Recalling our first face-to-face meeting, Mr Makita noted in his memoirs that he was struck by, "Mr Culver's appearance – as handsome as a movie idol, but possessing an air of decency and justness. Not overly aggressive, but nonetheless impressive." Mr Makita went on with this excessive praise, calling me "an attentive listener" who did not impose his views on others. Then came the age thing. Mr Makita said I was always very polite and constantly allowed him to take the initiative, seeing that he was about ten years older than I. Mr Makita recalled, "From time to time, he even made a joke of our age difference, referring to me as 'my father.' Sometimes I was even a little embarrassed by his persistent deferring to my view, but nonetheless, I appreciated his courteous treatment very much."

Mr Makita's approach was simple. He believed that the best way for us to improve relationships between Canada and Japan was to have Japanese businessmen meet Canadian businessmen face to face, so our major effort was to get as many people as possible to attend our meetings. One such conference in Vancouver had 450 participants, which was pretty impressive for that kind of event. And, out of those meetings came plenty of business for both sides. It was also thanks to Mr Makita that I was awarded the Grand Cordon of the Order of the Sacred Treasure, Japan's highest civilian decoration, in 1987.

It was because of my involvement with Canada-Japan relations that I had my only experience riding in a motorcade. They say if you ever do it once, you never get it out of your system, which may explain why politicians who get an official limousine seem to crave holding on to power so much. When Prime Minister Masayoshi Ohira died in office in 1980, Canada sent Governor General Ed Schreyer to the memorial service along with three other Canadian representatives. They included Bruce Rankin, who was our excellent ambassador in Tokyo, Quebec MP Charles Lapointe, and me. I presume that I was chosen because of my association with the Canada Japan Business Committee. On the day of the service, we were picked up at the front door of the Okura Hotel by the official motorcade, which sped us through the normally congested streets of Tokyo in no time. We arrived at the 15,000-seat Bodkin martial arts arena where the memorial service was being held and were greeted by the Japanese minister of foreign affairs. The four of us were among the last people to enter the hall, which was already full of mourners. We took our places in four tiny seats packed very close together. In the rows behind us, I could spot Imelda Marcos of the Philippines, looking as tough as nails, and Australian Prime Minister Malcolm Fraser, among others. Next to us were four empty seats. Two minutes later, the US group, led by President Jimmy Carter, was the final delegation to arrive. Carter was ushered to a seat adjacent to mine. It was so tight that I had my hands on my knees, and he had his hands on his knees, and our legs were almost touching. There was no room for lounging or stretching. Back in Montreal, where my wife watched the event on TV, she later recalled spending twenty minutes looking at my hand firmly gripping my knee because all the cameras were trained on the US president. Despite this instant intimacy, President Carter never uttered a single word to me or the three people sitting with him, including Secretary of State Edmund Muskie. He just sat and stared straight ahead. You'd think he would have said something, even the most cursory greeting. It was surprising to me that a politician could be so private in such a public setting.

As time went on, Canada's interest in Japan definitely waned, as the focus moved to China. Of course, Japan has been harshly criticized for its lost decade (1991 to 2000) after the bursting of its asset bubble, and there are some who now even talk of Japan's two lost decades. But when the history of the present period we're living in is written, we will probably talk about the current period when the economy stagnated in North America as a lost decade as well, and China will also probably experience the same phenomenon at some point. It's the old adage that what goes up must come down. It doesn't matter whether you're Japan, China, or the United States. It's true that Japan has a serious demographic problem, but they're starting to do something about it. There used to be close to five Japanese workers between the ages of fifteen and sixty-four in the labour force for every person over sixty-five. Now there are only 2.2. What they're proposing is a double-digit sales tax as the only way to deal with the fiscal shortfall. There is plenty of opposition to that proposal, but it may be the only solution to Japan's current difficulties.

In 1989, at my last press conference in Japan, when I finished my stint as chairman of the Canada Japan Business Committee, I was asked if I had any concerns about Japan. I admitted I was worried that it was going to be difficult for the Japanese people to accept China's emergence as a strong economy. In my mind, it was as much a psychological issue as anything else. I used to tell the Japanese that dealing with the United States is different than doing business with most countries because of Congress and how it works. I would tell them that when they had trouble with the United States, they should ask us Canadians for help. After all, the US is our neighbour and we have been dealing with the Americans since at least 1867. Although my Japanese friends and associates always treated the suggestion very kindly, they never once took us up on it. One day I said to my longtime friend Teruko, "Something strange happened today. During an official meeting of the Canada Japan Business Committee, the Japanese asked us to help them in their relationship with China! I was flabbergasted. They never took us up on our offer to help them in their dealings with the United States. Why in the world would they want our help with China, which is in their backyard?" Teruko answered immediately, "That's perfectly normal. We surrendered in 1945 to the United States without any conditions and they treated us very well. It would be improper for us to ever use an intermediary in our relations with the United States. But with China, it's not the same situation. You have many Chinese people living in Canada. Your Prime Minister Trudeau did a lot to help the Chinese get along in the world, so it's perfectly normal for them to ask for your help. But it would be improper for us to ask for your help with the United States."

The decade I spent promoting Canada-Japan relations almost led me to a radical career change as I was preparing to retire from Alcan in the spring of 1989. Brian Mulroney had called my friend and colleague Tom d'Aquino at the Business Council on National Issues and wondered whether I might consider accepting the post of Canada's ambassador to Japan. Tom, whom I knew extremely well, phoned me to sound me out. My immediate answer was, "Heavens no, I'm too young for the job!" Tom got a kick out of the answer, but in a society that venerates age it wasn't totally ridiculous. I was just about to turn sixty-five. The truth is that I wanted to start my own business, and I wasn't thrilled by the prospect of starting a diplomatic life halfway around the world and what that would entail for me and for Mary.

Although my primary focus was clearly on Japan in the 1970s and 1980s, I also knew that one couldn't long ignore China, even though it was still firmly in the grip of hard-line Communists and closed to foreign investment and global capital. Somehow, I knew this would change. Again, I was inspired by Alcan's history. Edward K. Davis had always felt that Alcan's next big aluminum smelter after Arvida would be in China, and he started to lay plans for that eventuality in the aftermath of the Second World War before the Communists seized power. We had a small manufacturing plant in China as early as 1934, and we were the last foreign company to be kicked out of China by the Communists in 1954. When I first went to China in 1978, one of the Alcan men who had worked at that plant twenty-five years earlier returned to see it. His report was that the pane of glass in the front door of the building that had been broken in 1954 was still broken in 1978. That was an example of the kind of progress that had been made in a quarter century of Communist rule. We were also selling ingot in China. In fact, I always knew when the bottom of the ingot market had been reached by watching the Chinese, who were great bottom-fishers. We were able to sell quite a lot of ingot in China in the early days.

The 1978 visit was organized by Paul Desmarais, chairman of Power Corp. of Canada, who had been urged by Prime Minister Trudeau to get Canadian business to take advantage of the political opening created by Canada's pioneering establishment of diplomatic relations with the government of Mao Zedong several years earlier. There were seven or eight leading businessmen on that trip, including Ian Sinclair, chairman of Canadian Pacific, Cedric Ritchie of Bank of Nova Scotia, Petro-Canada's boss Wilbert Hopper, and Robert Scrivener of Northern Telecom. We met with the Chinese leadership, and our work on that mission eventually led to the creation of the Canada China Business Council.

China in 1978 was still emerging from the dark days of the Cultural Revolution, a world away from the glitzy, prosperous China of today. All you saw were Mao uniforms, dull in colour and dreary in cut. Only babies and small children could be seen in brightly coloured clothing. The exception came one night in Beijing when we went back to our rudimentary hotel after dinner and got into the elevator. There we were, this group of big, tall Canadian guys, when a tiny Chinese woman got into the elevator. She was wearing her Mao uniform in exactly the same drab colour as everyone else, but you could see that it was made with a better quality fabric than the standard issue. The top button of her jacket was undone and the men, as we sometimes do, were all taking a little look. Underneath her jacket, the young woman was wearing a brilliant red silk blouse that was clearly very expensive. After she got out of the elevator, we all agreed that it was only a matter of time before those drab uniforms disappeared and coloured clothing returned.

Over the next five years, I returned to China three or four times. My attitude was that whatever Alcan would do in China, it should initially be small because we could learn as much about doing business in China with a small investment as we could with a big one. To get our toes wet, we eventually decided to build a small extrusion plant in Shenzhen, and to do even that we had to wade through a massive amount of bureaucracy. We needed 132 signatures to get that plant built, and each official seemed to be looking for something on the side before he would sign off on the project. When we refused to comply, they would offer to come to Montreal to give their approval, and we would politely reply that we would rather sign in Hong Kong or in Shenzhen. We finally got the plant built without paying off anybody, but thank God it wasn't a $100 million plant. It cost us maybe $4 million or $5 million at most. The experience confirmed for me the sense I had that it's natural for the Chinese to be commercial and build businesses, but not natural for them to let a business get to the point where it becomes bigger than what the family, including the in-laws, could manage. Once a business started to become bigger than the family could manage, they weren't interested in making it any bigger. That's why the Communists were able to build huge enterprises. However, in a non-Communist China, I've always had the impression that you wouldn't find huge capitalist businesses. That makes China different from Korea and very different from Japan.

In 1981, I was invited to travel to China with Henry Kissinger as a member of a delegation organized by the National Council for US China Trade that included eight US business leaders and Senator Bill Bradley of New Jersey. The Chinese leadership had asked Kissinger to advise them on what they should do to encourage foreign direct investment. We arrived in Beijing and were housed in their dreary diplomatic guesthouse, designed in a Cold War style that looked as if imported from 1950s Moscow. We boarded a small bus on the first morning and took off for an official meeting with Deputy Premier Bo Yibo. Bo was one of the "Eight Immortals," an informal cadre of Communist Party leaders who participated in the Long March with Mao Zedong. Bo was purged during the Cultural Revolution of the 1960s and thrown in prison, only to be rehabilitated after Den Xiaoping returned to power in 1978 and launched the country's capitalist-style economic boom. On the bus, I was sitting one row behind Kissinger, and during the ride to the meeting with Bo I leaned forward to ask, "When do we raise corruption and payoffs and, if so, with whom?" Kissinger replied "I am not sure if we do, but if we decide to, this is the man to do it with. He's the CEO."

The reception that day was formal if not stiff, and the seating arrangement reflected the atmosphere, with the foreign visitors on one side of a U-shaped seating plan, Kissinger and Bo side by side at the bottom of the U, and a bleacher full of Chinese bureaucrats enclosing the third side. After a fifteen-minute introductory talk by Deputy Premier Bo, Kissinger spoke briefly, and then Bo asked if we had any questions. There was a short pause, and then, to my horror, Kissinger turned to me and said, "Mr Culver has a question." I rose from my seat at the far end of our visitors' row, and, feeling somewhat uncomfortable and using lots of complimentary language, talked about my admiration for the progress China had made since my first visit in 1978. Then I added, if the objective sought by China was more investment from the West, something would have to be done about the rampant bribery and corruption that any investor meets along the way. I made it clear that I was hesitant to bring the matter up, but it was a real concern.

Bo replied carefully, laying out five points:

Do not hesitate to talk about corruption. We talk about it all the time.

We came to power because the Chinese people were fed up with corruption.

We have tried to get rid of corruption by making examples of offenders and using harsh punishments.

Our efforts have so far failed, so we must use laws.

But we have no laws and it will take time.

That was more than three decades ago. Now, as China's economy continues to rocket forward and the country is awash with new wealth, is the situation any better? There's probably no better answer than to look at the career of Bo Xilai, the son of Deputy Premier Bo Yibo, who delivered those reassuring words to me about China's anticorruption fight in 1981. The younger Bo rose quickly in the Party hierarchy, accumulated significant wealth thanks, in large part, to his father's contacts, and seemed headed for the top. But his career crashed after a headline-grabbing corruption scandal in 2011 that erupted after the death of Neil Heywood, the British businessman who had served as a fixer and middleman for the Bo family. Bo's wife, Gu Kailai, was charged and convicted of murdering Mr Heywood, and Bo himself was convicted in 2013 of bribery, embezzlement, and abuse of power and was sentenced to life in prison. Bo has been stripped of his membership in the Politburo and thrown out of the Communist Party amid promises by the new Chinese leadership that they plan to clean up corruption once and for all. Sound familiar?

8

"A Sense of Measure"

Multinational Musings

Business is business, and people are people, but one would have to be naive to believe that cultural, historical, and social distinctions between nations and peoples don't have a huge impact on the way you have to approach issues and get things done. For a company as geographically vast as Alcan, active in countries as diverse as Germany, Australia, and Guinea, it meant maintaining core corporate values like honesty and integrity while always remaining flexible to local concerns and ways of doing things. You had to be conscious that an approach that may have worked fine with employees at a smelter in Kitimat, British Columbia couldn't necessarily be transferred automatically to workers at an alumina refinery in Ireland or a fabricating plant in Uruguay.

And because of the nature of our business, which frequently meant steep capital outlays on facilities and heavy demand for electric power, governments and politicians were often key players who could not be ignored. That was the case even though Alcan always refused state handouts and never looked for political favours from the powers that be. That meant hiring good local managers who understood national and regional politics and could get us access to top decision makers if needed. Sensitivities to local conditions where we operated were always an essential ingredient to our overall success.

What being a multinational also meant was that Alcan was privileged to be able to capitalize on the skills of employees and managers from a host of nations and backgrounds who enriched the company with their diverse abilities and approaches. We may have been a Canadian company in terms of our headquarters and letters of incorporation but we were a global firm from our inception.

When looking at differences between nations, it's always instructive to analyze what I call their sense of measure. To give just one example, the reason for the inability of France and Germany to get along with each other for so many years in the nineteenth and twentieth centuries, with such catastrophic effects, was due to the fact that the French have an overly developed sense of measure, and the Germans have just the reverse. Germany is highly successful industrially because for them no issue is unimportant, which is part of their underdeveloped sense of measure. In industry, you have 1,000 things to get done in order to get a product out. In Germany, each task is as important as the other, which is why they make such exquisite cars and the world's best precision equipment. In France, it's just the reverse. While the French are good with the big picture, they drop the ball on the details. The problem is that the French have such a highly developed sense of measure they tend to get sidetracked to the point where the process being used to settle a serious issue becomes more important than the issue itself. Contrast that with a nation like Germany that does not have that same sense of measure. The Germans are very efficient because if they're faced with a problem they simply put their minds to solving it. They don't focus on the process that will be used to solve the problem. They just solve it. That's the industrial strength of Germany and of Japan as well. If I were an historian, I would try to write the history of modern-day Europe as a clash between an overly sensitive sense of measure and a less sensitive sense of measure.

In part because of their less acute sense of measure, Germans were always easier people to partner with than the French. Once I asked my first boss, Dr Haenni, who was Swiss, whom he'd rather be associated with – the Germans or the French. He responded, "I'd rather partner with the Germans because at least they'd admit that you're smart too. The French think that they're smarter than you are and therefore deserve more than 50 per cent of the partnership." To have a sense of humour, you have to have a sense of measure. You have to have the ability to laugh when you expect something small and you get something big, or when you expect something big and you get something small. It's the difference in scale between what you expect and what you get that makes you laugh. It's terribly important in life when you have to make a lot of decisions to have a view of whether you're dealing with something that's big or something that's not so big.

When I went around the world, one of the things I used to amuse myself with was finding out how much a country pays a comedian. A country that pays someone a lot of money to make them laugh is probably lacking somewhat in a sense of measure. A country like Britain doesn't pay comedians anything much. They make each other laugh and they're great at making fun of themselves. If Bob Hope had stayed in England rather than move to America, he'd probably have been a poor man. So a sense of measure is a great asset. Not only does it give you a sense of humour but it gives you the ability to make sensible judgments. And some nations are more blessed with it than others.

Britain has always been a key part of the company. It was in West Bromwich near Birmingham that Alcan installed its first-ever extrusion press in 1928, and soon the company was heavily involved in rolling sheet for the growing British aircraft industry. It was primarily with Britain's war needs in mind that the company undertook its massive expansion in the Saguenay during the Second World War. To assure an adequate supply of aluminum for the war effort, particularly for the construction of aircraft, Britain extended millions of dollars' worth of loans to Alcan, which were known internally as "the rubber notes." It was because of that cash inflow that Alcan was able to build the massive Shipshaw hydro-electric dam in the 1940s and undertake the related expansion of our smelting capacity. The structure of the rubber notes meant that when the war was over, interest and principal on the loans would only be paid in part if peacetime uses for the metal were not found for all this added aluminum output and the smelters were forced to operate at less than full capacity. As it turned out, this didn't prove necessary as aluminum consumption continued to grow for civilian uses after the war, and the emergence of the Cold War meant that military demand for aluminum soon recovered. In the end, these favourable loans were eventually paid back by Alcan ahead of time.

Alcan had built Britain's largest fabricating facility at Rogerstone in Wales, but when it came to primary metal, we continued to supply the U K with a lot of ingot from Canada for many years after the war. Foreign exchange was always a problem for the British economy, and in the late 1960s, Prime Minister Harold Wilson decided that, to improve its balance of payments, it was time Britain made its own aluminum with nuclear power providing the electricity. Three smelters, one in each of Scotland, England, and Wales, would eventually be built. Facing the inevitable, Alcan planned to build a smelter in Invergordon, Scotland, but for his own political reasons, Wilson didn't want Alcan to be the company to build that smelter. Rather, he favoured British Aluminium to do it. John Elton, who was running Alcan's operation in Britain at the time, decided that if Wilson would not let us build at Invergordon, we would put a power plant next to one of Britain's big coal mines, make our own electricity, and build our smelter right there. That put Wilson in a political corner because the smelter would be seen as supporting the coal industry, and the coal miners' union was still hugely powerful at the time, particularly with Wilson's Labour Party. That meant the prime minister could hardly say no to the project even though it wasn't linked to nuclear power.

We decided on a site in Northumberland in the heart of North-eastern England's coal country near the village of Lynemouth, which gave its name to the smelter. We paid for the construction of a new 420-megawatt power station, which took its coal supply from the nearby mine. We also obtained the right to sell any power beyond our own needs to the grid. The smelter opened in 1972, based on a twenty-year coal contract. But, the oil shocks of 1973 and 1979 meant that the contracted coal price was too low, and by the early 1980s the National Coal Board decided that we were going to have to pay a lot more than our contracted price for the coal to power our electricity plant. We were prepared to reopen the contract but not at their price. That led to a meeting with Mrs Thatcher, who had taken on the unions, including the once-powerful coal miners, but was still anxious to preserve the high-paying jobs that the Lynemouth power plant and smelter provided.

Mrs Thatcher had put Sir Ian MacGregor in charge of the Coal Board. He was a Scotsman who had worked in the US aluminum business before returning to the U K, when Thatcher asked him to run British Steel and then the National Coal Board. His goal was the same at both, to slash unprofitable operations and jobs and prepare both companies for privatization. We knew MacGregor from the aluminum industry and had great respect for him. When the Lynemouth coal issue was becoming acute, I ran into Sir Ian by chance in San Francisco, as we were both part of a crowd of people entering a conference hall. He said to me, en passant and not without a trace of a threatening tone, "You are going to pay a lot more for coal."

Lord Peyton of Yeovil was a longtime member of Alcan's board. A former Conservative M P, he had run against Mrs Thatcher for the party leadership but lost on the first ballot. Yet, he remained on good terms with the new prime minister and was named to the House of Lords in 1983, where he became one of Thatcher's major defenders. The managing director of British Alcan was Sir George Russell, a Briton who had begun his career with Alcan in Canada and had returned home as works manager of the new Lynemouth smelter. It was under Russell that Alcan had finally managed to merge with its chief U K rival, British Aluminium, after two unsuccessful tries. Russell had had a big role in the merger, and he was scrupulously fair in choosing the right managers from both companies to run the various divisions of the combined firm. Mrs Thatcher had named Russell to the board of the Civil Service Pay and Conditions Commission, so he was well known among

senior civil servants. It was thanks to Lord Peyton and to Russell
that I managed to get an audience with the prime minister herself
to settle this matter of the coal price once and for all.

All three of us arrived at 10 Downing Street at two in the afternoon. Walking in the front door, my first impression was that the
housekeeping wasn't very good and that the place was a bit frayed
at the edges. Mrs Thatcher's male secretary led us up the staircase,
past pictures of famous past prime ministers, warning us sternly,
"Now gentlemen, the prime minister has fifteen minutes, only fifteen minutes." We were ushered into the prime minister's office,
and it was spotless. Mrs Thatcher looked clean as a whistle, with a
slight scent of eucalyptus about her. She graciously invited us in.
"Oh gentlemen, come in and sit down over here."

She immediately started talking local politics with Lord Peyton
and George Russell. I don't remember what the subject was, but
she was going a mile a minute. Not a word about Alcan or coal. I
looked at my watch and twelve minutes had already passed. I figured that the guy from the colonies was going to have to be the
one to interrupt Mrs Thatcher because the two locals certainly
weren't about to. So I butted in. "Prime Minister, I'm sorry to do
this, but your secretary told us that we only have fifteen minutes.
We've already been here for twelve minutes and we haven't talked about what we came here for." "Fair enough," she responded.
"What's the problem with coal?" I said, "The problem with coal is
that we signed a twenty-year contract before the oil shock, and the
current price is obviously too low. We're prepared to pay a higher
price but not the price being asked. I have to tell you that I run a
company in Canada that doesn't take subsidies from government,
and we're not here to ask for a grant from your government. All
we're here to do is arrange for a fair price under the circumstances." Then she asked me "Well, what do you think is a fair
price?" I responded, "Well, it so happens that most of the coal that
comes out of the Ellington mine is sold to Sweden. We'll pay
whatever Sweden pays less the freight, because with us there is
no freight. We use the coal right on the spot." She turned to her
secretary and declared, "Fix it." Then, without missing a beat, she

turned back to Peyton and Russell, "Now, as I was saying, gentlemen ..." And, we were there for another half an hour or so discussing British politics, having gone way past the fifteen minutes that the secretary had insisted was our limit. It was clear she had made up her mind and wasn't going to waste any time making small talk about coal pricing.

I met Mrs Thatcher again in Vancouver a few years later during Vancouver's Expo 86. Lord Peyton had heard that she was going to meet with a group of about a dozen senior businessmen of which I would be a part, so he spoke to the prime minister's staff and told them that I would be there. When it came time for the reception, I stood at the far end of the receiving line. When Mrs Thatcher got to me she said, "Oh, Mr Culver, how nice to see you again!" as if we were old friends. Lord Peyton had done his job.

Dealing with politicians was certainly not my favourite way of solving issues, but maintaining cordial relations with presidents, prime ministers, and ministers was simply part of the job, and, on issues like the British coal contract, it did allow for quick and definitive solutions to thorny problems. It also permitted me to meet some of the most fascinating leaders of the time. Michael Manley, the charismatic prime minister of Jamaica was such a personality. Jamaica was home to a large bauxite and alumina operation that was an essential part of Alcan's supply chain for its Canadian smelters, particularly after Guyana nationalized Alcan's bauxite operations there in 1971. Although there was no imminent threat of expropriation, Jamaica was also caught up in the anti-colonialist rhetoric and leftist politics that had infected much of the Caribbean. Manley was friendly with Pierre Trudeau but also was playing footsie with Castro in Cuba. As president of Aluminum Co. of Canada, part of my remit was Jamaica, but I didn't know quite what to expect when I went down to Kingston to meet Manley in the mid-1970s.

I had heard a lot of good things about his father, Norman Manley, who had been Jamaica's prime minister from 1959 to 1962 and was fondly remembered by a lot of the old Jamaica hands at Alcan. As I walked into Michael Manley's office, I wondered to myself whether he was as good a man as his father had been. The prime minister held out his hand and said immediately, "Mr Culver, I'm pleased to meet you, and I want you to understand that everything I know, I learned from my father." He had evidently read my mind. Manley was a real charmer, and it was hard not to like him. He was keenly aware that Alcan had already been kicked out of Guyana by its socialist prime minister Linden Forbes Burnham. Anxious to broach the issue of Alcan's future relations with Jamaica, I suggested to the prime minister that he might like to buy out our bauxite and alumina operations in Jamaica at book value if he didn't like the way we were running them. "Oh no, my friend Burnham told me never do that," Manley said. "Don't ever buy them. Just tax them to death." Manley was admitting that Guyana's plan to become rich after nationalizing Alcan's mine hadn't quite gone according to plan. What Burnham hadn't realized when he nationalized Alcan was that he had only taken over one link in a chain, and, consequently, Guyana had given up all connections to that chain. The only people who would buy Guyana's bauxite after 1971 were the Russians who paid him 15 per cent less than he had been getting from Alcan.

Yet Manley's threat to jack up our taxes, even delivered with such seeming bonhomie, wasn't exactly a reassuring answer. Clearly sensing my unease about his ultimate goals, Manley got straight to the point. "I suppose you're afraid that I'm going to turn Communist." I thought I owed it to him to be just as candid in my response. "Well, I've thought about it, I must admit," I said. Manley continued, "Let me tell you something. Do you know what a higgler is? Higglers are what we call those Jamaican ladies who sit by the side of the road and sell you a piece of fruit or a bottle of Coca-Cola. They are the ultimate small traders. Do you think it would ever be possible to turn people like that into Communists?"

The Jamaican alumina plants were always tricky to manage. They required skill to run because of the way they were built and the chemical characteristics of the bauxite they were using, but the Jamaicans had the skill to do it. As Jamaica's major foreign exchange earner, along with tourism, Alcan was an important economic presence on the island. We led the way in remediating exhausted bauxite mines and turning them into productive agricultural land, simultaneously becoming the island's largest milk producer. I once said to Mr Manley, "You know, I like Jamaica a lot and I have a lot of fun when I'm here, but you guys are the Irish of the Caribbean." He was taken aback. "No one has ever said that to me before. What do you mean?" I responded, "Well, you're like the Irish in that when you go abroad you're hugely successful. Jamaicans do very well when they leave Jamaica. But as long as they stay in Jamaica, all they do is fight with one another, which is a very Irish habit."

When I visited Jamaica, I would typically stay at the managing director's house that Alcan owned near Mandeville, a charming town with a distinctly English feel that was close to our main bauxite operations. On staff at the house was a chauffeur named Marcus, as conservative a man as you'll ever meet. On one occasion, as he was driving me through Cockpit Country, a rugged forested area of inland Jamaica with narrow, winding dirt roads, Marcus asked me, "Do you know why the roads in Jamaica are so twisted?" I replied that it must have something to do with the geography of the place. Not at all, responded Marcus, "It's because we didn't used to have cars. We only had horses. And Jamaican horses are lazy. If you put a Jamaican horse on a straight road, he'll say that he can't make it to the corner. But if you put him on a twisted road, he can always make it to the next corner."

The close friendship of Manley and his wife Beverley with Pierre and Margaret Trudeau certainly didn't hurt our bilateral relations. I'm convinced that personal relationships count among world leaders, even as they do in business. I have no doubt that when Obama meets Putin or Harper, there's a desire to be friendly, and it's always easier to deal with issues of substance when there's a good human rapport. George Shultz, the former US Secretary of State and a very wise man, once told me that the Cold War began to end when Gorbachev and Reagan had their first meeting in Geneva in 1985. As usually happens prior to these summits, both he and Reagan had been scripted by hordes of diplomatic people as to what would happen when the meeting took place. According to Shultz, when the two leaders first met, Reagan broke the ice with a story. "I understand that speeding is a big problem on the streets in Moscow, and the police have strict orders to ticket anyone who gets caught, no matter how important they are," Reagan told the Soviet leader. "From what I hear, one day you were running late for a meeting. Concerned about being on time, you told your chauffeur to get in the back so you could drive and get there faster. Minutes later, two policemen stopped the limousine for speeding. One of them approached the car but didn't give you a ticket. When his colleague asked him why he let the car and its passenger proceed, the cop responded, 'Too important.' His colleague was perplexed. 'Who was it?' The first cop replied, 'I didn't recognize the guy in the back seat but he must have been important because Gorbachev was driving!'" The joke worked like magic. The meeting led to a subsequent summit in Reykjavik, Iceland, and from then on the bureaucrats on both sides lost control of what Gorbachev and Reagan were going to talk about.

I headed Alcan in the final years of the Cold War and stepped down just months before the collapse of the Berlin Wall, which touched off a series of huge political and economic changes including one that had a major impact on Alcan. Russia's huge aluminum industry, which had been essentially outside the world trading system, was soon privatized and its output unleashed on international markets, with huge implications for the pricing and supply of the metal. As it turns out, the Alcan I left on 1 July 1989 proved to have been much easier to lead than what was waiting for my successors!

While I missed that shock, I was around for the earlier emergence of Australia as a powerhouse in the aluminum business. For Alcan, Australia was for many years a bittersweet story. We had started there, as we did in many markets, by sending ingot from Canada to Australia, before the war. An Australian company called Comalco had built a small smelter in Tasmania, and when it came up for sale at one point, a colleague in Montreal made a strong plea for Alcan to buy it. But we didn't buy it, which was an error. A much bigger mistake occurred a few years later when an Australian prospector arrived in Mr Davis' office at Alcan headquarters and said, "I have discovered bauxite in Northern Australia, excellent bauxite which has Alcan's name on it." Mr Davis said, "I think you're right, but we're in the middle of building Kitimat right now, and we're up to our eyeballs in expenses, so I'm afraid that we don't have the money to buy it." On his way home to Australia, the prospector stopped in San Francisco and sold the project to Kaiser Aluminum, which ended up developing the Cape York bauxite mine. That was the second opportunity that we missed in Australia.

The third one occurred a few years later when our own geologists discovered bauxite on the western coast of Australia. That bauxite wasn't as rich as the bauxite from Cape York and had lower alumina content. This new Australian discovery was also not as rich as the Boké deposit in Guinea, which Alcan had decided to make into its bauxite priority. Because the Australian ore was lower in value, Alcan figured it wasn't worth shipping it all the way to Canada to process into alumina and then into metal. When Alcoa looked at the deposit, they saw the same economics but decided not to ship the bauxite anywhere and to produce alumina right there in western Australia, which was the correct decision. All this turned Australia into a major producer of bauxite, alumina, and aluminum, and its proximity to booming markets in Asia, particularly China, have served it well. In the end, Alcan missed three major opportunities in Australia. Moving ahead to 2007, one effect of Rio Tinto's purchase of Alcan was to eliminate two of those three major missed opportunities because the takeover finally brought both the Cape York bauxite operation and Comalco into the Rio Tinto Alcan fold.

Though we may have lost out on a few Australian business opportunities, Alcan took full advantage of the availability of talented Australian managers. They were a great bunch. Australians have this appealing combination of the British sense of humour and the American sense of informality. They don't take themselves quite as seriously as Canadians do and are certainly more fun loving. Some of the Australians whom I originally got to know were in family businesses and were accustomed to seeing their fathers take annual business trips to England. Travelling by ship, they would be away for nine weeks at a time. When air travel came along, these Aussies saw nothing wrong with flying to England but still found a way of making it into a nine-week trip. They convinced Qantas, the national carrier, to take a more interesting route to London than the conventional one, which had stops in Honolulu, San Francisco, and New York. Starting in the 1960s, Qantas began operating the "Fiesta Route," which flew from Sydney to Tahiti, then on to Acapulco, Nassau, and finally London. The flight was scheduled only once a week, so my Australian business friends would spend a week in Tahiti, a week in Acapulco, a week in Nassau, and then on to London where they finally got to work.

When I first went to Australia in 1957, it was pure white. You hardly ever saw a face of a different colour anywhere, which was particularly striking because Australians were all alone way out there in the Pacific. Since that time, the country has become much like Canada. Australia has accepted immigrants from all over the world and is now a much more heterogeneous society. It's a great place to live if you have money to fly out of there when you start feeling isolated. Excellent weather. Next to Montreal, Sydney would be my first choice if I ever were to move.

New Zealand was even more British than Australia. You felt as if you were one hundred miles off Land's End in a place populated by displaced Londoners. To give you an idea of the atmosphere, the first night I arrived in New Zealand in the late 1950s I was locked out of my hotel because I had stayed out beyond the hotel's 9:30 p.m. curfew! And the food was as awful there as it was in Australia. They used to say about Australia and New Zealand that, "a balanced diet is a meat pie in each hand." But, these days the food in Australia and New Zealand is world-class, thanks in large part to those new immigration policies.

Brazil soon joined Australia as a centre of bauxite mining, alumina refining, and smelting. Like Australia, it had abundant resources and a can-do mentality that was refreshing. Brazilian managers are excellent, and the Brazilian people are graced with a sense of humour, which is the same as saying that they have a good sense of measure. They are blissfully free of complexes. In my days in Geneva, one of the lecturers was the great French geographer, André Siegfried, who had the Frenchman's ability to talk without notes and then start reading some notes without his voice changing in tone. (Every time an English person switches from speaking off the cuff to reading, his tone changes.) And, Siegfried's notes were something else. He had probably been using the same penciled scrawls for his lectures for a generation. His presentation to us was on North and South America and their heritage as multi-racial societies that had emerged out of slavery, immigration, and large indigenous populations. "In North America, if you have one drop of black blood in you, you are black," Siegfried told us. "In South America, if you have one drop of white blood in you, you are white." It was an atrocious generalization, yet there was an element of truth to it. One of the reasons I love Brazil is that there's no element of colour consciousness at all. They accept people from other countries who, from then on, regard themselves as Brazilians. In contrast, Argentina would accept British, Germans, and Italians who would then regard themselves as British living in Argentina, Germans living in Argentina, and Italians living in Argentina but not as Argentinians. Argentinians seemed to have trouble adopting a national identity, whereas Brazilians seemed to adopt theirs naturally.

The upshot of this was that we could use Brazilian managers anywhere in the world, although at times it was hard to move them because of the high quality of life they enjoyed at home. I once asked a young Brazilian to come and work in Montreal at Alcan headquarters. He declined. "It would be a nice promotion," he conceded. "But in Brazil I live first class. In Canada, even you don't live first class."

Alcan's experience in Venezuela was nowhere as positive as it was in Brazil. We tried to do business there, but we discovered quickly it wasn't going to work for us. I would argue that there is something about Venezuelan culture that is not very appealing. They have a custom in Venezuela in which, during carnival season, Venezuelan wives and sweethearts dress in black masks and go out on the town to settle personal scores. The men pile into the bars and drink a lot, at which point the disguised women arrive, and it all gets very nasty. I decided that this was not a nice society. We had a partner in Venezuela who was somewhat unique. We flew down on Alcan's plane to see him and make a deal. When we landed in Caracas, our aircraft was unexpectedly given Gate #1 at the airport, with a Pan Am plane on one side and a Varig Airlines plane from Brazil on the other. When the plane door opened, the first person we spotted was our potential partner. "Come with me; our car is right over there," he told us. We piled into a van that had benches along the sides with a table in the middle on which a bottle of vodka on ice had been strategically placed. We never saw anyone from Customs or Immigration and drove straight out of the airport. In the car, our potential partner introduced us to Venezuela's former president, who had just been voted out of office. We drove up to our associate's fancy house, on a hill above the teeming city, and were marched through the house and out to the swimming pool. And, using words I'll never forget, he said, "Mr Culver, this is my swimming pool, and you can pee in it if you want to." I thought to myself, "Who are these guys?" Needless to say, we ended up not having a very fruitful relationship with him.

The Venezuela example emphasizes the importance of being very selective in your choice of partners and agents if you're to avoid the dangers of bribery and corruption. If you once give in to corruption in the slightest way, the flood gates will open. Your only choice is to say that you don't do it and accept the consequences. That can be hard, particularly in the case of petty corruption, sometimes called facilitation payments. Take a customs officer in an Indonesian seaport. His salary is probably no more than US $100 a month, so he makes his living by taking small payoffs for signing the papers that get the goods through the port. If you are operating a manufacturing plant in the country and a key piece of equipment that makes the whole thing work is being held up at the port unless a palm is greased, do you pay or not? It's a real problem. What many companies do is to hire a local lawyer or agent who's the one who greases the way. To be honest, I don't know if we had a lawyer who occasionally paid. I remember sitting on a flight beside an American man on a trip back from Indonesia, and he said that he had gone to his lawyer and asked him what to do in just such a situation. The lawyer told him, "Go and call on the customs agent at the port, and while you're talking to him, reach down and pick up a wallet off the floor that has 50,000 Rupiah in it. Hand it to the agent and say, 'I think you dropped this.'" He told me that he played the game in similar circumstances. When he reached down and picked up the wallet, which he had brought with him, and gave it to the customs agent, the agent checked the contents, and said, "That can't be my wallet because my wallet had 100,000 Rupiah in it!"

I remember when we sold our South African holdings, and we were congratulated by the good lady from an antiapartheid church group who had attended all of our annual meetings. After the meeting, I said to her, "Why didn't you ask why we got out of twelve countries in Africa and not just South Africa? If you want the truth, we stopped doing business in those twelve countries partly because of cost, but also because we couldn't be there and not engage in local corruption."

Like other developing nations, India was also challenging for Alcan, but we managed to build up an excellent business there including an extensive fabricating operation. We had solid Indian partners and excellent Indian management, including a wonderful managing director named T.D. Sinha. He was a very serious-minded, upper class Indian gentleman who had amazing patience with the bureaucrats who are so powerful in India. I could never understand how he did it. I guess he'd grown up with them, and he just accepted how they worked. India's bureaucracy had this strange approach to capitalism that involved placing obstacles in front of successful firms. They believed that if you were better than the rest in your industry it would be unfair to the others to let you grow. Alcan would ask for permission to make a modest investment of $4 million to $5 million to improve the output of one of our plants plant by, say, 10,000 tons a year. The bureaucrats would inevitably say no because they insisted it would put our competitors at a disadvantage. I used to refer to the Indians as millions of greyhounds on a leash.

The chairman of our Indian company at one time was Field Marshall Sam Manekshaw, a former chief of staff and a national hero because of his brilliant leadership of the Indian Army in its 1971 victory in the war against Pakistan. He first made a name for himself as a highly decorated officer in the British Army during the Second World War and remained sprightly, quick, and slim decades later when he joined Alcan after his retirement from the Indian Army. He was more British than the British, once telling a journalist that upon waking at 5:30 every morning he liked drinking a small glass of whiskey, listening to the BBC news, and puttering in his garden before going to work. On one of my visits to India, Field Marshall Manekshaw took Mary and me on a one-day tour of some sights, ending up at Agra, home of the Taj Mahal. During our tour, we stopped for lunch at a small hotel somewhere in the countryside, and the staff was very impressed to be serving India's most famous soldier. One of the staff asked their illustrious visitor, "Field Marshall, could I offer you a scotch?" He replied "Young man, I never drink before 6 p.m., and I seldom stop thereafter!"

I once went to see Prime Minister Jawaharlal Nehru in the late 1950s or early 1960s. India needed aluminum, and Alcan had spare ingot for which we couldn't find buyers. I offered Nehru a deal on 5,000 tons of aluminum ingot on very favourable payment terms. Nehru looked at me and in effect told me to go back to Prime Minister Diefenbaker and tell him that if he knew what was good for him Canada would give India the aluminum free of charge. That was the end of that. A few years later, I went to Delhi to try to get government permission to pay a dividend from our Indian company. The answer from the deputy minister in charge was a categorical no. It was impossible, he said. There would be no foreign exchange provided to Alcan for a dividend. I told him that if

we couldn't take out a dividend in cash we'd have to take it out
on the hoof. Perplexed, he asked me what I meant. I said that we
would just take our best Indian managers and use them in other
parts of the world, which we did and there was no objection to that
from the authorities.

Though I loved visiting India, the bureaucracy could be exhaust-
ing and exasperating, but its idiocy occasionally provided comic
relief. At one point, before Alcan bought its Challenger business
jet, we decided to test out how owning one would work for us and
borrowed Inco's Gulfstream II, which was a pretty fancy plane in
those days, to fly us to India from Montreal. After our last meeting, we headed to Bombay Airport. We could see the Gulfstream
sitting on the tarmac just outside the terminal building, but it took
us an hour and a half to get to it. Corporate jets weren't exactly
common in India at the time, and the authorities didn't know how
to handle them. Before we could even enter the terminal we were
asked for a boarding pass, which of course we didn't have. After
negotiating around that issue, we had to go through customs and
immigration, and at that and every other step of the process, offi-
cials kept phoning Delhi for various permissions. All the time,
Mr Sinha, our local managing director, was with us, remaining
very patient. We seemed to be finally through all these formalities
and approached the door to walk out to the plane. Just then, a big,
strong man with a crooked smile and straight teeth blocked our
way. He asked in a loud voice, "Crew?" I immediately said, "Yes!"
and we marched right through. We were about to take our final
steps to the plane when another official yelled, "Stop! You can't
walk across the tarmac. You have to ride!" So we had to wait until
they brought out an airport vehicle to take us the few hundred
yards across to the plane. We got to the bottom of the steps where
the Inco pilot was standing in his uniform, looking impatient and
extremely irritated. We started up the steps, and the pilot leaned
over and said, "Dave, if you ever want to come back to this fucking
place, you'll have to fly the plane yourself. I'm not coming back
here again." I asked, "Did you have a hard time?" He responded,
"Yes. I could only change $240 worth of travelers' cheques at a

time to buy fuel. So I've been spending two and a half hours going back and forth buying $240 worth of fuel so we have enough to get us to Bahrain." That was Indian bureaucracy. We flew to Bahrain and then to Shannon late in the evening, where the contrast couldn't have been greater. There wasn't an Irish customs officer in sight. We were told that they were all in the pub. Someone asked us whether we would be leaving the next morning. When we said yes, they responded that it was fine, so off we went to our hotel without ever seeing a customs officer. Such was the contrast between India and Ireland.

9

"Like A Trip to the Kennel"

Growing People

My first proper job interview was certainly unusual. It was with Dr Paul Haenni, who was running the Centre d'Études Industrielles, Alcan's business school in Geneva. He wanted to see if I was interested in staying on after the end of my studies there to help run the school as a member of staff. His first question to me was a bit of a zinger. "Young man, do you have a motto?" To be honest, I had never thought of adopting a personal motto, but I had just seen a quote in an old copy of the *Reader's Digest* that seemed as if it might just do the trick. "Nothing in excess, even moderation." That's my motto, I told Dr Haenni, being careful to avoid telling him its distinctly unintellectual source. He seemed to like it. Then he asked me whether I knew what the three secrets of happiness were. I had done pretty well conjuring up a motto on the fly, but I had no further inspiration so I asked Dr Haenni for his view. Dr Haenni replied with his three secrets to happiness.

Take pleasure from small things.
Always have an alternative.
Set reasonable near-term goals.

Three simple pieces of advice that I immediately committed to memory and have relied upon all my life. Taking pleasure from small achievements or tiny luxuries makes the difficult attainment of those often illusive big goals so much more tolerable. Having an alternative means that you don't end up being cornered by a situation simply because you've been fixated on one solution and never contemplated any other possibility. And by setting reasonable near-term goals you don't start off your career by saying, "My goal is to become C E O of Alcan." Instead, you figure out what your goal for the next week is and do something specific."

When I was working with Alcan's sales team in New York, I was still too junior to have any responsibilities for hiring and firing, but I observed the hiring practices of others, figuring out what seemed to work well and less well. It was only when I returned to Montreal in 1956 that I reached the point where I had to start making decisions about hiring people. From the start, I have never been a great believer in choosing new employees simply on the basis of C V s. It's true that C V s are useful for getting the basics and leading to further questions. They save time because you don't have to ask people where they've worked previously, where they did their studies, and all those other background details, but they give an incomplete picture. My first advice on hiring people came from a lecturer at the school in Geneva, a wonderful man called Colonel Lyndall Urwick, a Briton who was one of the original management consultants. I remember him expounding on his theory of personnel recruitment. "You know, there are all kinds of scientific tests and tricks that you can use," he told us, "but it all comes down to something like a trip to the kennel. You can do all the research in the world before choosing the dog you want, but you can't avoid getting to the point where you have to look down at the dogs in the kennel and decide which one you want to take home with you. You can't get away from the personal contact and the gut decision as to which of the dogs you think will make the best companion." It's the same with people. Anyone who hires simply on the basis of consulting a C V is crazy. So an interview is essential. Or, a game of golf.

You learn a lot about people on the golf course. For one thing, you discover whether they cheat, even a little bit, and whether they can control their feelings. It's a rare golfer who can hit a bad shot and not comment on it or hit a good shot and not boast about it.

When it comes to cheating, I think that many golfers do it. They nudge the ball when they think you're not looking, or they press the dirt behind the ball with their foot while talking to you in the hope of giving the ball a better lie. In the end, golf is a test of your physical and mental self-control and a great test bed for future employees.

Taking Colonel Urwick's advice, I always made sure to meet a prospective hire in person. My own approach was to interview a job candidate one on one for at least thirty minutes and sometimes have the people with whom they would be working interview the candidate as well. When I became Alcan's CEO in 1979, I needed a chief personnel officer. It was a key position. First of all, I knew it had to be somebody who would be accepted within the company as nonpolitical and fair. Secondly, it had to be somebody who would stand up to me and tell me straightaway if they thought I was doing the wrong thing and explain why. Not everyone in an organization has the presence of mind and gumption to tell their boss that he's doing something wrong. I had heard about a fellow named Roger Maggs who was running a small plant that Alcan had in Uruguay, and my instinct told me that he would make a good HR guy. The problem was that we had never met. I was going to Brazil on business, and since I knew he was in the general neighbourhood, I asked him to meet me in Rio. This rather short fellow, looking very British, bounced into the lobby of my hotel. He was wearing some kind of well-tailored, dark blue blazer with brass buttons, a Cambridge tie, and all the rest of it. I broke the ice with an easy question. "Well Roger, tell me something about yourself." And he responded exactly this way: "Well, my wife is a medical doctor, and she tells me that I'll never grow up." Very droll, self-deprecating, and with a marvellously outrageous sense of humour. I figured that any guy who's being interviewed for a huge promotion and tells the interviewer, who happens also to be the CEO, that his wife believes he'll never grow up, must be a guy who's not afraid to tell the truth under any circumstance. I hired him, and he ended up being absolutely first class even though he had not an iota of HR experience before getting the job. He was a real person who could deal with the strengths of people and their weaknesses. The chemistry was right, and I knew from the start that he wasn't going to bore me. I think you have to work with people that you enjoy being with. After all, you spend plenty of time at work and it should be something you look forward to rather than dread.

Roger Maggs went on to other senior positions at Alcan in metal marketing and mergers and acquisitions before leaving the company to cofound Celtic House, an Ottawa-based venture capital firm. His founding partner in Celtic House was fellow Welshman Terry Matthews – they came from the same town in Wales – who happens to be one of Canada's most successful high tech entrepreneurs.

A lot of people would say that I took a big risk by turning to an operating guy from a small subsidiary in Latin America and transforming him into the top H R officer at headquarters even though he had no substantive prior experience in personnel. My response is that it may be great to look for experience that's relevant to a position that needs to be filled, but you have to be careful that it doesn't turn into a trap that stops you hiring the best person for a job. It may sound a little harsh, but the art of management is learning how to get first-class results out of second-class people. Not second class in a bad sense, but hiring or promoting people who may not be ideal and allowing them to grow into a position. Looking for the ideal person for a specific job is not likely to get you nearly as far as finding a way to take a less than ideal person and let him succeed. If I had to describe my job as C E O in a single phrase, it would be "to grow people quickly." That's what I once told Myron Kandel who interviewed me on Lou Dobbs' show on C N N. His initial questions were very friendly, but towards the end of the interview he lobbed me the following hot potato, "Well, Mr Culver, if you had to describe your job as C E O of Alcan in one sentence, how would you describe it?" I knew he was expecting to hear me expound in detail about adding shareholder value, increasing earnings per share, and all that stuff. Instead I said simply, "My only job is to grow people quickly. If I can grow the people working with me quickly, they'll push the company up."

In searching for an example of growing people, it's instructive to look to the late Paul Desmarais, the longtime chairman of Power Corp. of Canada and an old friend of mine who passed away recently. He established a large personal estate at Sagard, an isolated place in Quebec's Charlevoix County, hardly a sophisticated locale with a wide range of skill sets to choose from. The Sagard estate is extensive and a very complicated place to run, but most of the main jobs are held by people from the tiny town adjacent to the property. What Paul did was hire the world's best golf club manager or golf course superintendent, bring that person to Sagard for six months to teach his skills to a locally-engaged employee. At the end of the six months, the job was handed over permanently to the local person who had just got all this fabulous training. This process built an excellent cadre of highly skilled employees with a commitment to the job and the employer. It's also one of the reasons that the Desmarais family is so well thought of in the community.

When hiring, I think that there's value in using headhunters, provided that you use them in a judicious and task-limited way. That's easier to do with a headhunter than it is with McKinsey & Co. or any of the other high profile management consultants. My theory on management consulting is based on the premise that it's possible to run a successful business and do ninety-eight of one hundred things slightly wrong, provided that you do the two essential things absolutely right. On that theory, management consultants make a fortune by telling C E O s, "Do you realize that you're doing ninety-eight out of one hundred things slightly wrong?" The C E O agrees and says, "Help me fix it." In the process of working on the ninety-eight slightly wrong things, the consultants manage to screw up those crucial two things that the company has done absolutely right from the start. With headhunters, the task is more specific, and they can be highly useful, especially when you turn to the international firms with their extensive inventory of extremely competent individuals. However, in most instances, you should try to promote from within before looking outside. It's very hard for people to feel that they're gaining traction in their company or organization unless the business is growing and that the people they work with are advancing. Even though seeking new blood can be the best solution at times, always looking outside for talent is a sure way to discourage your most ambitious and most competent managers.

Even with the help of headhunters and all the best hiring practices imaginable, on occasion you do end up with the wrong person in a job. You're only human, and you're going to make mistakes, so it's best to move quickly to try and correct the damage. What you don't want to do is let a situation smoulder. It's not fair to any individual or to the organization as a whole to do that.

One of the traits I think is most useful in a good manager is one that may seem counterintuitive and can be hard to detect in a job candidate, particularly when they come in from the outside. I believe that good managers are big talkers. In a world where discretion is often seen to be at a premium and companies spend millions to protect their intellectual property and corporate secrets, this may seem to be a strange character trait to value. After I left Alcan, I was told that I was often referred to as a blabbermouth. Why? Because when I was facing a problem I would describe it and talk about it with anybody in the company. I'd tell my chauffeur on the way home that I had a problem and be genuinely interested in what he had to say about it. It's human nature in large organizations to regard knowledge as a source of power and, as a result, not to share it. The theory is that you know something that the other guy doesn't know, so you're more powerful than he is. That may protect your own little patch of territory, but it does nothing toward solving the company's problems and moving forward. In my mind, good managers lay it on the line for everybody to see and work as a team to solve problems.

My predecessor as Alcan's chief executive, Nathanael Davis, was not what would be conventionally known as a blabbermouth. Far from it. He was not a voluble person and was actually quite shy, but Nat would always tell me everything that I needed to know to get my job done. He never rationed information, unlike what is too often the case in large organizations. What really gets my goat is the kind of manager who gives intelligent people an assignment without telling them the key bit of information. It is as if they were participating in some sort of elaborate party game. That's the sort who returns to the manager, who has been working extremely hard on the assignment, and says, "You forgot something." That something, of course, would be the key bit of information held back in the first place. This kind of game is simply a waste of time and also smells of elitism.

I learned a lot from Nat, but he did have one little habit that really irritated me. If he didn't like somebody who was working for me, and usually it was for a question of personal behaviour rather than for a business reason, Nat would pick a time when I wasn't around and fire the guy. It happened on at least three occasions. I had one man working for me who was a genius but difficult to handle, and, to be honest, with a lifestyle that was a bit free and loose. Nat, who was extremely straitlaced, fired him when I was out of town. Ironically, after he was fired, this same man stayed in the aluminum business and ended up becoming a very good customer of Alcan. Another time, when I was in the hospital for a hernia operation or something similar, I got back to work to discover that Nat had fired one of my guys while I was convalescing. It was during another hospital stay that Nat got together with Dana Bartholomew, the chief financial officer, and transferred a guy who was working for me. They not only moved him out of my group but they put him in charge of another fellow who was also working for me, and I knew from the start that those two would never get along. Yet, I knew that once Nat had decided, there was nothing to do about it. It became a frustrating pattern. On one of these occasions, I heard about Nat's little surprise on a Friday afternoon as I was headed to Lake Manitou for the weekend. I was still stewing about it after I drove up to the lake and actually thought of quitting. I woke up on Saturday morning and told myself that I had to do something to relieve the tension, so I phoned the local farm supplier and ordered a load of manure. I asked him to dump it on the front lawn. I spent the rest of the weekend transferring the manure into wheelbarrows and spreading it over the lawn. Shovelling that truckload helped me deal with my frustration and did wonders for the grass.

This annoying quirk of Nat's HR approach aside, I learned immeasurably from him. Above all, I learned decency and how to take the long-term view. He taught me how to let people complain short-term, provided you were convinced they were going to do the right thing long-term. Nat tended to run Alcan a little like it was a family business. The beauty of a family business is that you have no shareholders harping about every quarter's earnings, which allows you to run the business patiently, focusing on the longer term as well as the short term. I am proud to say that in all my years at the company and despite its status as a leading public company, Alcan never forecast earnings. That was E.K. Davis' rule, and I followed it assiduously, to the frustration of journalists and financial analysts alike.

Alcan had an unusual history as far as its CEOs were concerned. In the early years, Edward K. Davis ran Alcan out of an office on Newberry Street in Boston, even though the bulk of the operations were in Canada and most management was based in Montreal. When Nat took over from his father in the late 1940s and Alcan was still growing, he continued to run the company out of Boston. He was supported there only by a secretary and one or two additional staff. It was a pretty original way of running a multinational before the days of email, video conferencing, and other forms of instant communication. The rest of the Alcan executive offices were located in New York in a low-rise building at Rockefeller Center just across from Saks Fifth Avenue. A separate sales office for the ingot business, where I worked in the early 1950s, was located nearby in Rockefeller Center on the twenty-sixth floor of the British Empire Building just behind the giant statue of Atlas. One day several years later, after I had relocated to headquarters in Montreal and was back down in New York for a visit, Nat and I and Eric West were standing on the corner of Fifth Avenue and 54th Street after a dinner at the University Club. I turned to Nat and told him, "I really think you should be in Montreal. That's where all the people who work for you are and I think that you should be there with us." Eric, who was a longtime Alcan colleague and dear friend, disagreed, convinced that Nat would be overwhelmed by the move and killed by the pressure. I can't say that my advice was the prime motivator, but Nat did move to Montreal a short time later in 1962, about the time we moved into Place Ville Marie.

It may sound curious but even during those years of running the company from Boston, Nat and his senior managers never seemed to feel isolated from Alcan's operations in Canada, staying in touch by Telex, telephone, and mail. In the early days, there were also frequent overnight train trips to Montreal. Mr MacDowell, my boss in sales, actually lived in Rhode Island. He spent weeknights at the University Club in New York and his weekends at home in Rhode Island. And then there was Dr Earl Blough, the original technical man at Alcoa and later Alcan as well, the inventor of some of the very first alloys that were used in aluminum. As vice president responsible for research, exploration, and engineering, Dr Blough worked in New York but lived outside the city. Long after he had retired, I ran into him one day on Fifth Avenue in New York. He must have been more than ninety at the time, a man who was small in stature, very perky, and with quick movements. "Dr Blough, what are you doing in New York?" I asked. "Oh," he responded, "I come into the city every week for a haircut and a dance lesson!"

When Nat moved to Montreal, he created a management committee of about fifteen senior people who decided on all the big issues facing the company. I was all in favour of sharing information, but I found it excessive that a group of fifteen was needed to make a decision. It slowed things down, which became an issue as competition increased and we at Alcan and other producers no longer controlled the price of aluminum, then being set at the London Metal Exchange. We had to move faster. When I became CEO, I still shared the same information with everybody but ensured the final decision was made by four or five people. If anybody had a different view, our doors were always open, and it was their responsibility to make that view known.

Perhaps I picked this up from Nat Davis, but I was never a hugely stressed out person. Between Friday evening and Monday morning, I would forget what Monday morning was going to be all about. I didn't bring work home, and I even made a point of not bringing my pipe home in the days when I was smoking a pipe. If on occasion I took home a large briefcase, I usually wouldn't open it. To some, that might be considered slacking off, but I firmly believe that everybody needs some down time. While nobody could ever accuse me of being a workaholic, I did have some workaholics working for me. I also had micromanagers around me who would wear themselves out. I myself was much too lazy to be a micromanager. If you're a micromanager, it's a terrible burden to run a big organization. One of the stories told about Jimmy Carter's presidency is that his aides and other employees weren't allowed to use the White House tennis court unless they first got Carter's express approval on the day they wanted to use it. What exactly was the president of the United States doing controlling the use of the White House tennis court?

Closer to home, Jacques Bougie, who became Alcan's C E O several years after I retired, was a highly talented manager who burned himself out by being a micromanager. When David Morton became C E O after me in 1989, he named Bougie as his number two and put much of the work on Jacques right from the start. As a result, even before he became C E O himself in 1993, Jacques had been carrying a big load for four years. As time went on, it became clear that the pressure of the job was getting to Jacques. I was skiing at Mont Tremblant around that time and bumped into him in the tow line. His eyes were glistening. This man was clearly under an awful lot of pressure. Eventually Jacques went to the board and submitted his resignation. He simply couldn't take the pressure. Having saved himself by resigning as C E O, Jacques has remained active in the business world as a corporate director and dedicated himself to new responsibilities in the nonprofit world. He has done a fabulous job as cochair of the Montreal Neurological Institute's fundraising campaign, proving that he had all the qualities I originally recognized in him as a successor at Alcan.

Being able to delegate is not only important to save your own sanity as a CEO or other kind of leader, but it's also important if you want good people to work for you. If you can't show people that you trust them, it's not going to work. It's a key part of growing people and growing them quickly.

Delegating is important, but it doesn't remove the responsibility of a leader to be aware of the big picture. The way I kept track of whether the business was going well or not so well, whether we were going up or down, was to keep mental track of unexpected events that occurred during the day. I kept a balance sheet in my head of the number of unexpected events that were helpful versus the number that were hurtful. If one exceeded the other, it would indicate the direction in which we were going.

One of the essential qualities I would always look for in a manager is character. By that I mean selflessness, which also means learning how to listen. Great leaders are good listeners, and they know that good ideas can come from anyone and anywhere. Some leaders excel at running an existing organization, but very few can actually change an organization. Many CEOs could have run IBM, but only a Lou Gerstner could have changed IBM. And, he did it not simply by having a clear vision of where he wanted to take the company; he did it by listening. Wise people become good listeners and work hard to remain so.

I've always worked on the principle that in an organization there should be very few solid lines. A solid line represents the power and the ability to give an order if necessary, and as such it works in one direction only, which is downwards. The guy at the top of the line can give an order to the guy at the bottom but not vice versa. While I believe there should be few solid lines in any organization, there should be infinite dotted lines. With a dotted line comes the responsibility to give advice whether asked for or not at one end of the dotted line. At the other end, the responsibility is to ensure that the person who gives the advice understands and accepts what you do with it. Dotted lines work both ways and there should be dotted lines between every single person in an organization. The key to success is a multitude of dotted lines, and you have to remember that to make these dotted lines work, you have to be a good listener.

As in marriage, selflessness is essential to being a successful leader. I believe that too much ego can get in the way of being a great leader. When I retired from Alcan in 1989, Patrick Rich was the most obvious person to succeed me. He had achieved a lot at Alcan and was extremely effective. He also had a kind of charisma. In fact, he had a lot of Trudeau about him. He was a Frenchman from Alsace Lorraine, a polyglot, and a citizen of the world. His father had fought for the German Army in the First World War and for the French in the Second World War. Patrick himself had degrees in political science, European studies, and law from Strasbourg University and had also been a Fulbright scholar in economics at Harvard. In addition to French and English, he spoke German, Spanish, Italian, and Portuguese. After serving in Algeria with a French paratroop brigade, Patrick joined Alcan as a project analyst and later worked for the company in Africa, Europe, and South America as well as in Canada. To top it all off, he could have become a first-class professional jazz pianist. In fact, when he was working for me I had to spend some of my time scheming to keep Patrick from jumping ship and getting involved in the music business. Adding to Patrick's charisma was his personal style, including his penchant for wearing long black leather coats. He was a lot of fun to be with. The name Rich ended up being a bit of a nuisance for such a well-travelled man, after the financier Marc Rich fled the US for Switzerland and became a wanted man. Patrick used to get stopped and held at many borders until authorities assured themselves he wasn't Marc Rich.

But despite this charisma, and perhaps he had just a bit too much of it, I did not choose Patrick as my successor at Alcan. I'm a strong believer that great leadership requires great selflessness and not selfishness. When he was passed over for the top job, Patrick left the company and in the ensuing four or five years he first became C E O of a large Swiss private company and then C E O of British Oxygen, a big public company. All the while, I sat in Montreal wondering whether I'd made a terrible mistake in not naming him as my successor. In the end, there was just too much ego there. That worry remains with me today, but it is eased by my continued friendship with and liking of Patrick. He has done well for himself and his family, is satisfied with his accomplishments, and remains my envy at the piano.

Roger Phillips, who ran Alcan's Canadian smelting operations in the 1970s, had a high IQ and understood engineering problems extraordinarily well. He was an outstanding man. He was opinionated and wasn't afraid of expressing his views whether taking on the unions or criticizing governments. But all this meant that he did have a certain edge to him that at times I found inappropriate particularly within the Alcan organization. I used to tell him, "Roger, there's only one person in Alcan that you can be rude to, and that's me. If I catch you being rude to anyone else, you're out of here." In the end I had to let him go from Alcan for just that reason. But Roger had an impressive career after he left. He went to Saskatchewan where he took over the leadership of the steelmaker Ipsco and built the company successfully over the next twenty years. He and I remained very friendly up to his death in 2013, but I still believe that if Roger had demonstrated a bit more graciousness he could have gone to the top of Alcan. Whenever a colleague left Alcan, I used to say, "The only way you can do Alcan harm would be to not be a success in your new job." Both Pat Rich and Roger Phillips did Alcan and me proud.

As a boss, I never saw the point of yelling or being abusive. It wasn't in keeping with my personality, and I never thought it was a very effective form of management. One result of this approach is that I don't think people were particularly scared of me, although I never saw this as undermining my authority. I can only remember twice in my career when I let my temper get the better of me. In one case, I walked out of the room in the middle of a meeting, and the other time I hung the phone up on somebody. After the second incident, I happened to see John Nichol, a member of the Alcan board and onetime Liberal senator from British Columbia. "John," I told him, "I did something today that I've never done before. I slammed the phone down on somebody." He responded

"David, don't do that. Here's what to do next time you feel the same kind of frustration. If you just can't stand dealing anymore with a particular phone conversation, you say, 'Now look here, there are three reasons why I' – and press the button on the phone to end the call. That way the person on the other end will just think that he got cut off." On the other occasion, when I walked out of the meeting, I was particularly annoyed and just couldn't take it anymore. I left the office and went home. I remember not feeling very well about the situation, so I lay down on my bed and sent one of the kids to get me a glass of brandy. It shows you how out of character it was for me to walk out on anybody. It literally made me feel sick.

One reason I never took an aggressive approach to my job as CEO is that I knew the limits of my authority. When I was young and had no clue where my work life would lead me, I used to think how nice it would be to eventually become a chief executive. I figured that once I got the top job, I would be able to do whatever I wanted, and nobody would be able to stop me. It didn't quite work out that way. The higher I rose the more I had to do what others expected me to do. I discovered that I had to constantly learn how to compromise. I realized that being CEO was primarily about doing what was possible and not just what caught my fancy at any particular point in time. Being a successful leader is doing what is expected of you while at the same time working to achieve your own vision of the future. You can only attain that goal by being selfless and not by cracking off and doing whatever you want to do. That's the art of leadership. A good leader also recognizes that any large organization needs a variety of skill sets. The best description of those skills came to me from a man named James T. McCay, an extraordinary individual who was an expert on time management, a consultant to big companies, and also a motivational speaker. A graduate in engineering from University of British Columbia, he worked as a petroleum engineer in the Persian Gulf before transforming himself in the 1950s into an executive trainer and early management guru who founded a firm called Integron Associates. He was a tall, imposing man with a shaved head and who invariably became the centre of attention the moment he entered a room. Always dressed in a long black silk jacket and matching silk trousers, he wore a large metal pendant around his neck that supposedly represented the essence of Integron, whatever that was. Such was McCay's personality that he seemed to consume whatever young woman was sitting at the reception desk as he arrived at Alcan's office. I can still remember him coming to see me the day after I was named head of Aluminum Co. of Canada in 1975. He told me not to get carried away with myself. "Lots of people can run Alcan," he told me. "But few can change it."

McCay's theory was that within any company, there are four types of individuals: the hunter, the spiritualist, the court jester, and the leader. Taking his cue from prehistory, McCay described the hunter as an individual who believed that the only way to keep the tribe alive was to hunt an animal and drag it back to feed his kith and kin. Within a company, the hunter thinks in pretty simple terms like, "All this business needs is more sales." The spiritualist approaches the activities of the firm in terms of right and wrong and then asks, "Is this what we should be doing? Is this ethical? Is it moral?" Then there's the court jester who, to alleviate tension in a business situation, will inevitably crack a joke or say something to get everyone back to being productive again. The final type is the leader. According to McCay, the only reason he's the leader is that, of all four types, he is the only one who knows why you need the other three to succeed. Recognize these types. Go through any group or company with which you are associated, and you'll find them. While the world may seem to be in constant flux, human nature is the one thing that doesn't change.

Good CEOs whom I've encountered also know the technology of their business inside out. They understand and have the ability to define and think about their customer's business. A good leader who knows not just his customers but, more importantly, knows the needs of his customers' customers is the one who succeeds.

Rather than centralize decision making in the large management committee that Nat Davis had set up, I placed more emphasis on area managers, each of whom was the boss of everything that was Alcan in his particular region. But, when it came to technology, I thought that it was essential to share expertise across the company, so I created peer groups in key sectors of the business. Take the case of rolling mills. I would take the best rolling man in each of the areas worldwide and have them meet. A leader would emerge from those meetings, the top Alcan rolling man of all the experts we had in that field. Under that arrangement, it was his role to approve every significant rolling mill investment that we built anywhere in the world. The Alcan expert in that field was a German, Reinhold Wagner, who ran our huge rolling mill in Norf, Germany. I wouldn't approve an investment in rolling equipment anywhere in the world unless Wagner had studied it, been to the region, and said it was the right thing to do. I found that having these peer groups meet regularly was a very efficient way of making sure that our technology was up to scratch all the time. The strategic decision of whether we added more capacity at a facility or shut it down would be taken by the area manager as part of his responsibility for day-to-day operations. However, if the man in charge of Latin America felt that it was time to build a really big, new, modern rolling mill in Brazil I would want Mr Wagner to assure me that what was being proposed was the right thing to do.

But I didn't want all decisions to emanate from headquarters. When I joined Alcan, there was a boss of operations worldwide, an amazing guy called Mel Weigel. From his office in Montreal, he would fire off a missive to India telling a mill manager that he should move a piece of equipment from building A to building B. That kind of micromanagement can only be carried off by a uniquely qualified individual. Mel once accosted me when I was a young salesman. "Culver, when are you going to stop selling what the customers want and start selling what I want to make?!"

I've always felt that managing a growing company is the ideal because managers and employees all feel as if they're contributing to an enterprise that's progressing, and it means that there are always new opportunities for ambitious people. When economic circumstances turn against you and cutbacks are essential, the challenge is greater and maintaining morale becomes really tough. The recession of the early 1980s was particularly punishing to the aluminum business, leading Alcan in 1982 to report its first annual loss in many years. Production was cut, and prices were awful, so we had to take action. The first thing I did was to cut my own salary and directors' fees by twenty-five per cent and ask all senior managers to work for two weeks without pay. Then I cut all nonunion salaries at the company by ten per cent, although I exempted all employees with salaries at $50,000 or less. In addition, I asked all the nonunion staff, including those with lower salaries, to work an extra thirty minutes a day and left the choice to employees whether it would be added on at the beginning of the day or at the end. The new work day became 8:30 to 5 or 9 to 5:30. The main thing in this kind of situation is to be very open and to talk to everybody frankly about why these kinds of decisions are being made. At the time, I had to tell some very decent and loyal employees that presence at work is not necessarily value at work. We have office hours because of interdependence, but never having been late getting to work for twenty years does not in itself make you invaluable!

This extra effort in tough times was accepted with equanimity everywhere within the Alcan family around the world with one notable exception, the Saguenay region of Quebec. I got a call from the provincial minister of labour telling me that I was offside and couldn't ask people to work an extra half hour a day. It was a question of *les droits acquis*, acquired rights. In the end, the only people at Alcan who refused to work that extra half hour a day in the midst of the toughest recession since the Second World War, were those located in the Saguenay. And, by the way, none of them lived more than fifteen minutes from work, so the extra half hour was hardly going to create a disruption on the home front. It was simply another case of Quebec exceptionalism.

Young people often ask me how to assure success in their career, how to make it to the top. I try to remind them that you don't have to be excellent all the time. You only have to be excellent at the right time. That's why, when I was hiring people, I tended to hire those that were good at sports. Whether they realized it or not, they were usually the kind of people who had mastered the trick of being right at the right time, not necessarily struggling to be right all the time.

Another trick to knowing exactly when the occasion calls for excellence is to learn how to capitalize on the inevitable. I once asked a man who was working for me in Washington DC to explain how to work most effectively with the US government. His advice was to follow three golden rules. First, always pay attention to what is going on around you and capitalize on the inevitable. Second, always stay in with the outs. In other words, spend your time with people who are not in power. The people who are in power now may not have time for you while everyone is seeking their attention, but those who are not in power have time galore to spend with you and, most importantly, they will eventually be in power. So, stay in with the outs. And the third one was never, ever get between the dog and the tree.

And, I would add, never ignore happenstance. By happenstance, I mean the occasions when something seemingly irrelevant happens. It may seem irrelevant but the wise person wonders why it happened. "Maybe I should pay attention. It's telling me something." These are essential elements to acquiring wisdom and preparing the mind for what may come. Wise people tend to be happy people. They tend to follow fairly reasonable practices and reasonably good policies. Occasionally, wise people may be wrong, but they maintain open-mindedness towards happenstance and miracles. Follow that, and you may well find it makes you a wiser person. Chance favours the prepared mind!

10

"An Outsider on the Inside"

The Trials of the Independent Director

Being an outside director, particularly of a large corporation, may sound like a wonderful job for somebody who loves business but doesn't want the day-to-day headaches of running a massive organization with all that it entails. After all, you get to hobnob with the great and the good, often in the loveliest of locales, the hours aren't bad, and you actually get paid for doing it. I was particularly privileged to serve as an outside director on the boards of many great multinational companies including Seagram, American Express, and American Cyanamid as well as several other firms. But after years of loyal service, I concluded that it's a nice honour to be an outside director but not much fun. To be honest, very few outside directors were actually ever effective, not more than fifteen to twenty per cent of them.

It's extremely difficult to be an effective outside director. It all comes back to what General Doriot taught me at Harvard Business School. Every business organization consists of a whole lot of people helping one person do a job. Outside directors end up being part of the same group that includes the company's officers and top employees who are there to help that one person, the C E O, do a job. The only difference between an outside board member and all the others is that the outside director also has the onerous responsibility of changing the C E O if required. Basically, the outside director is in the untenable position of helping and supporting the C E O but also being around to sack him or her if necessary.

There's a real conflict there. If, as an outside director, you consistently acted as if you wanted to change the C E O you would in effect be pulling the rug out from under him, which is exactly the opposite of helping him. You would be hurting him. Yet blindly following that C E O even when he or she is pursuing the wrong course for the company is not an acceptable alternative either. The trick is to choose the right moment when you switch from being one of the gang that's helping the C E O to being one of the gang that wants to turf him out. That is a skill that few of us learn to master.

It all starts with the fact that in most companies the outside directors are chosen by the C E O. If a C E O approaches you and asks you whether you would consider joining his or her board, the first thing you should ask yourself is whether you're prepared to help this person. "Do I think the person is good enough, and am I prepared to be one of those who are there to help him or her?" If the answer is yes, then the first time you think that the C E O is doing something wrong you naturally hesitate to speak up about it. When I was an outside director and saw that the C E O was doing something dodgy, I'd look around the boardroom, and usually discover that no one else was complaining. In a fast-moving world, you knew that the C E O had probably already committed himself to the decision you didn't agree with. He might have said that this or that proposal had to go to his board first, but usually he'd already committed to a course of action before consulting the directors. When nobody uttered a word in protest, I would say to myself that I might as well sit back and do nothing. What I would then do was go home and write the C E O a letter. I'd say very politely, "You know that deal we approved the other day? I don't think it's good for the company. I seemed to be the only one in the room who was feeling that way, but let me tell you why I don't think it's a good deal. I realize it's done now, so the matter is over as far as I'm concerned, but for future reference this is why I don't think it was a good deal."

A year later, another issue would come up, and again I would feel uneasy. I would look around the room and, once again, would realize quickly that no one else was going to speak up. This time, I'd go and see the C E O in person and be very transparent, which very few people were willing to do. I'd say, "You know, you'll recall that I wrote you a note a while ago and said that I thought you were doing the wrong thing. Let me tell you again why I think you're doing the wrong thing." If it happened a third time, it was clear that the time for silence around the table had ended. I would turn to some of the other directors and say, "Are you happy with this? Maybe we should have a discussion." The end result of that was usually a pretty messy situation where the C E O ended up getting turfed.

You were putting yourself through all of this for a director's fee that was usually not that fabulously high anyway. Too often I would suggest something to the C E O at a board meeting and he would thank me but then do nothing with my suggestion. Then, two months later, I'd learn that the company had hired McKinsey & Co. or another management consulting firm to advise them, and lo and behold, after a big fee had been paid, the consultant would tell management the same thing that I had told them. This time the company would follow the advice. A much higher fee was paid for the same advice I had offered.

Despite what sounds like carping on my part, I did love to participate in most of the boards I served on because of the people I met and the places I went. The board of American Express was a case in point. It was loaded with nineteen of the world's most fascinating and accomplished individuals. I'll never forget my first American Express board meeting in a huge room with a big round table at the Amex headquarters in Manhattan. American Express had a novel approach to these meetings, notably a seating plan. Most companies don't have a seating plan, and people usually end up sitting in the same place, next to the same board member at every meeting, like high school students at lunch in the cafeteria. But Amex would change the seating plan at every meeting, to mix things up. It's a formula that I liked.

At my first Amex board meeting in 1980, I found myself seated next to Gerald Ford, the former president of the United States. The meeting began and Jimmy Robinson, the Amex C E O, was going a mile a minute on some complex financial maneuver that he was contemplating. In the middle of all this, President Ford turned to me and said, "Do you understand what he's saying?" I said, "No, I haven't got a clue." So Ford stuck his hand up and said, "Jimmy, stop right there. There are two of us over here who don't know what you're talking about." I thought that was such a nice way for him to make me feel at home. Gerry Ford was a wonderful guy, with no pretensions.

We also had Henry Kissinger, who had a noticeably droll sense of humour, on that board, and we also had a man I really loved, Bill Bowen, who had been president of Princeton University as a younger man and then ran the Andrew W. Mellon Foundation for many years. And there was Vernon Jordan, the former US civil rights leader and adviser to Bill Clinton, who's also a great guy, Beverly Sills, the opera singer, and Frank Popoff, the head of Dow Chemical. We also had a fellow named Charlie Duncan from Texas who had inherited a coffee business that was subsequently bought by Coca-Cola in the days when Robert Woodruff still ran Coca-Cola. (Duncan also was US Secretary of Energy under President Jimmy Carter.) When Coca-Cola took over Charlie Duncan's company, Charlie was invited to join the Coke board. One worry he had on joining the board was that Woodruff was getting old, and it was unclear what Coca-Cola was doing to find a new C E O, particularly because Woodruff was such a dominating – in fact domineering – character. But Charlie's mind was set at rest at his first board meeting when Woodruff announced that he was going to step down from all his positions at Coke as of the following April. Furthermore, Woodruff told the board he was going to nominate somebody else, let's call him Adams, to take over. Charlie was relieved. The April meeting came and Woodruff stood aside, ceding his place as chairman and C E O to Mr Adams. At the next meeting, the new chairman and C E O was firmly in place at the table, and Charlie thought to himself that this was going pretty well, considering his earlier fears. But, at the following meeting, there was no sign of Adams. He had disappeared from the picture. Charlie turned to Woodruff and asked, "Where's Adams?" Woodruff responded, "He's gone. The son of a bitch thought he was running the place."

It was while I was on the American Express board that I witnessed and participated in something that happens only rarely at big publicly owned corporations, a board led movement that resulted in the resignation of the long-serving C E O, James D. Robinson III, whom we all knew as Jimmy. He was an exceptionally talented individual, with a great eye for others with talent, and forcing his resignation was not a decision that was obvious or easy for the board. This was not an overnight event. Far from it. What finally undermined Jimmy's standing with the board was a long and painful series of decisions that hurt the company with financial analysts and the market. The theory behind many of those decisions was one that I, for one, was suspicious of from the start – that customers of a financial services firm would value "one-stop shopping." Before the arrival of Visa and MasterCard, major retailers like Eaton's in Canada and Saks Fifth Avenue in the US provided clients with their own store-branded credit cards. My mother appreciated the way this enabled her to buy everything she needed at Eaton's with considerable convenience. Hence, the idea of one-stop shopping. But, once she had a Visa card that was accepted widely she used Eaton's less and shopped wherever she wanted. Would it be any different with financial services?

The other thing that bothered me about Jimmy was that he believed strongly that the main purpose of American Express was to increase earnings by fifteen per cent annually year in and year out. At one board meeting, he and Sandy Weill, his number two at Amex at the time, made a presentation to the board outlining this philosophy. I timidly raised my hand and said, "Somehow or other, I don't think business works that way. I don't see how you can say that you're going to do that no matter what the business cycle is." Coming from a business background where commodity cycles ruled, I had trouble believing that the only way was up, based on a simple mathematical goal. Their response to me was clear. "Well, that's the way we're going to do it." The first board member to raise the question of a replacement for Jimmy was Rawleigh Warner, the former chairman of Mobil Oil. A veteran Amex director, at seventy-one he was nearing the mandatory retirement age for directors. I received a message to contact him, and when I called I found myself talking to Mrs Warner. She told me that her husband wanted to arrange a meeting of outside Amex directors to discuss the C E O's position. I said that I would attend such a meeting, but only if Jimmy were present as well. Her response was one of surprise. "Are you kidding? You want Jimmy to be there while you discuss replacing him?" I replied that as a former C E O myself, if the same thing had happened to me I would have liked to be present. In the end, I don't recall that meeting ever taking place. I think that the first time we formally discussed Jimmy's future was at a subsequent board meeting after he had left the room. In the heat of the key meeting when the decision to replace Jimmy Robinson was taken, I slipped out to the bathroom. Just then, Henry Kissinger walked in and said to me in his deep, heavily German-accented voice, "I thought I was a student of revolution. I've never seen revolution like this!" Jimmy's replacement was Harvey Golub, a very competent guy who had been number two at the company but represented a major cultural change for a W A S P y white-shoe firm like Amex. Harvey wasn't in the job for long before he began strongly urging his successor should be Kenneth Chenault, an African-American. Ken, who's a lovely man, became C E O in 2001 and is still there.

Soon after Harvey had replaced Jimmy Robinson, Amex stock started rising from the twenties into the thirties. When it hit somewhere around $33 or so, Amex got a call from Warren Buffett saying that he would like to buy ten per cent of American Express. He had already started accumulating the shares through his holding company, Berkshire Hathaway Inc. We had about 500 million shares outstanding at the time, so ten per cent was fifty million shares. At $33 a share, that meant a lot of money, even for the Sage of Omaha. Buffett was asked. "Would you join the board if you got that ten per cent?" To which he replied, "No, I can't join the board." When Buffett was asked how he would vote his shares if he got his

ten per cent, his answer was straightforward. "As long as Harvey
Golub is the CEO, I'll vote with the board. Change Harvey, and I
reserve my rights." So he was willing to bet more than $1.5 billion
on one guy. By early 1995, Buffett disclosed that he had amassed a
9.8 per cent stake in the company or 48.5 million shares. The shares
later went up to $100, and Buffett made a ton of money. It comes
back to my fundamental principle that the board's main job should
be to find the right person as CEO. One of Amex's moves during
the Jimmy Robinson days was the purchase of Shearson Lehman
Brothers. While on the Amex board, I was appointed to the
Lehman Brothers board and made chairman of the Compensation
Committee. If there ever was a case of a chicken being put in with
the wolves, it was I at that moment. There I was, a guy from a conservative, small-town company like Alcan being put in charge of
the Compensation Committee for a Wall Street banking firm. The
experience only confirmed my long-held belief about investment
banking, which is summed by one basic premise: Wall Street
investment firms should be partnerships only; they should not be
public companies. Partners should be playing with their own
money not with shareholders' money, and it's when investment
companies go public and forget this premise that they get into
trouble.

At one of the first Compensation Committee meetings that I
attended at Lehman, I was presented with a list of nineteen names,
each representing someone who was due to get a bonus of more
than $1 million. What was curious is that I didn't recognize a sin-
gle name on that list. I had never heard of any of them.

That group of nineteen didn't include the top people at Lehman,
who had already received much bigger bonuses that had been
approved by the American Express board. I said that I wanted to
meet these nineteen people and was told that wasn't necessary.
I insisted, so a meeting was reluctantly arranged. I told the nineteen, "Look, I'm being asked to approve your bonuses, and I think
I know how the system works. I know that I have to approve them,
but let me say one thing to you: this is January. If in July I find that
some or all of you are asking American Express to put more

capital into Lehman Brothers so that you can do more business, I'm going to ask you each to put up half of your bonus as your share." The response was angry. "Oh, that's not the way it works," I was told. I continued. "Well, maybe it isn't the way it works, but I'm trying to make a point." In any case, I didn't remain chairman of the Lehman Brothers Compensation Committee for more than a few months after that. All these years later, I still believe that the investment banking business is critical to a well-functioning capitalist society, but investment banks should be partnerships and not public companies.

That brings me to a subject that's the rage in management schools and beyond these days, the issue of governance. There's a whole generation of professors and well-meaning book writers who have made a career out of preaching about good governance. I personally think that the governance issue has been over-stressed. It is important, but it's not all-important. Directors should focus their attention on how to find and nurture the right CEO. On a scale of one to ten, I'd give governance a rating of about five. But I'd give getting the best CEO possible a rating of 9.9 out of 10. All business is about helping one person do a job. If you need a board to instil good governance in a corporation because the CEO isn't creating it himself, you've got a problem. It's at that moment that the directors should put their collective foot down. The thing about the governance craze is that a lot of money has been made by consultants and authors writing about good governance, and I would bet that some of the people who have written these books don't actually practice good governance themselves.

It's hard enough to be an outside director in a big, widely held corporation. It's more of a challenge when the company is controlled by one group, particularly a family. That was the case at Seagram, where I served on the board for almost twenty years. The Seagram board was essentially a rubber stamp. One of the things that Edward K. Davis insisted on for Alcan was that Alcan should never have a director who had a business relationship with the company. Never name your lawyer, your corporate banker, or your investment banker to your board. If they're doing business with the company, they're not on the board. That was his rule. The Seagram board, by contrast, was chock-a-block with the company's lawyers and bankers. How can you get honest advice from people whose livelihood depends on staying on the good side of senior management?

My biggest regret as a director of Seagram was agreeing to Edgar Bronfman Jr.'s questionable decision to sell Seagram's twenty-five per cent stake in DuPont. Shortly before I joined the Seagram board in 1982, the company made an unsuccessful bid to buy control of Conoco, a big oil and gas company. Seagram lost out in the battle to DuPont but still ended up with a significant chunk (32 per cent) of Conoco, which it later swapped for the twenty-five per cent stake in DuPont. At first glance, the transaction appeared like a loss for Seagram, which had tried and failed to buy all of Conoco. Getting twenty-five per cent of DuPont may have looked to some as being the booby prize. In fact, it was just the opposite. If Seagram had managed to win its original bid, Conoco would have been into Seagram for $300 million in cash a year to finance its extensive oil exploration operation. Seagram traded its stake in Conoco for twenty-five per cent of DuPont, which provided them with a dividend of $240 million a year. In one fell swoop, Seagram had a $540 million annual cash swing.

After Edgar Sr. anointed his son Edgar Jr. to take the helm of Seagram, the old way of doing things at Seagram was doomed. Edgar Jr., a sometime songwriter and film producer who had spent lots of time in Hollywood, was clearly enamoured with the entertainment business. Yet nobody on the board, and I include myself in that group, made a peep to object to the purchase of Universal Pictures or to the eventual sale of the company's cash cow, its twenty-five per cent stake in DuPont. At the mumbling level, Charles Bronfman was against it, and Leo Kolber, the longtime Bronfman family confidant who headed the family investment firm, was against it as well. Yet, when the sale did come up before the board, I found myself arguing in favour of the deal. I admit to making a couple of mistakes. The first is that I bought into Edgar Jr.'s argument that, as good a company as it was, DuPont was unlikely to outperform the s & p 500 over time. He used that argument to explain why he should be allowed to sell DuPont and spend the money on Universal Pictures. The second mistake I made was that I read Edgar Jr. as being somebody who would be extremely good at running a movie studio and the music business. What I missed was that there was not one other person in the whole Seagram organization who knew a thing about films or music. It would have been like Alcan going into the casino business on the basis of a single senior executive's whim.

There were plenty of signs that Seagram was losing the Midas touch that the founder, Samuel Bronfman, had shown in growing the business over decades. In the early 1980s, Seagram made an unfortunate plunge into the business of mass-market table wine. At one of my first board meetings, Edgar Bronfman Sr. stood up and proudly introduced a young, attractive woman named Mary Cunningham who had been recently hired as Seagram's vice-president of strategic planning with special responsibility for expanding the company's wine business. When she was hired, Ms Cunningham was a 29-year-old Harvard M B A who had come to public attention after her ultra-rapid rise as an executive at Bendix Corp. and her subsequent departure. After sifting through 170 job offers, according to her own account, Ms Cunningham finally ended up at Seagram where she gave us a typical Harvard Business School Marketing 101 presentation on why Seagram should get into the table wine business.

When we broke for lunch Edgar asked me, "What did you think of Mary Cunningham?" I responded, "Well, she's obviously smart, but how does she stack up wisdom-wise?" borrowing the phrase I had first heard thirty years before from those Madison Avenue advertising guys at my gin-on-the-rocks lunch. Edgar wondered what on earth I meant. I said, "Frankly, I think it's a dumb idea. There are two brothers in California named Gallo. They're in their seventies and they're worth a billion bucks apiece." Edgar was always a bit earthy, and in fact some of the best off-colour stories I've ever heard came from him, so I knew I could get away with what I was going to say. "Edgar, if you and your brother were in your seventies and worth a billion dollars each, I'm sure you would rather protect one percentage point of market share than have an orgasm! The Gallos are not going to like Seagram plunging into the table-wine business, and it's not going to be profitable." Edgar disagreed, and Seagram ended up paying $237 million for Wine Spectrum, a subsidiary of Coca-Cola with several wine brands that Coke seemed happy to dump and which Seagram sold a couple of years later.

When at a board meeting Edgar Jr. first raised the subject of going after Universal Pictures, I said, "Edgar, I have a question for you. Are you getting bored with the booze business?" "Oh, no!" he replied. "It's a wonderful business!" I went on, "Make sure you're not getting bored with the girl that brought you to the dance." Edgar's response was to go and buy worldwide distribution rights to Absolut Vodka to show that he wasn't bored with the booze business. Of course, he wasn't really interested in the alcohol business even though it had been the basis for his grandfather's great fortune. I later told Leo Kolber that one of my deepest regrets was that I didn't speak up against this disastrous series of decisions for Seagram. Leo said to me, "Don't hold it against yourself. There was no way you were going to stop it anyway. None of us could have stopped it." Overall, few people on the Seagram board spoke up against these moves, and that ultimately led to the demise of a legendary Canadian company.

While being an outside director in a family-controlled company meant accepting certain constraints, it was nothing like being a director of a government-controlled corporation. I served on the boards of both Atomic Energy of Canada Ltd and Canadair Ltd, the aircraft manufacturer, when both belonged solely to the Canadian government. For those of us serving on those boards, the dreaded phrase we would hear from time to time was "the shareholder." Whenever the deputy minister appointed to the board stood up and commenced a statement by talking about the wishes and desires of "the shareholder," we would cringe. We knew that meant that the government in power wanted Atomic Energy to build a heavy water plant in some depressed region of the country, even though the company clearly didn't know what to do with the planned output. It didn't matter because Atomic Energy wasn't really being run as a business. It was being run as an instrument of public policy. That made it difficult for the businessmen who were on the board to understand and see what the point of their participation was. The corporation had major problems finding foreign buyers for the Candu nuclear reactor, but that wasn't really surprising since, outside of Ontario, it was next to impossible to get Canadians to buy it. How were we expected to sell Candu reactors abroad if Canadian provinces wouldn't buy it? When I finally left the Atomic Energy board, I must admit to being thoroughly relieved.

In general, though, what I found most frustrating about serving as an outside director was the fact that as board members we were usually presented with matters for discussion which in many cases were a virtual fait accompli. We tried to do things differently at Alcan, but not everybody liked our way of doing things. When Jack Welch was appointed head of General Electric, I picked up one of the guys who had been passed over for that job, John Burlingame, to join the Alcan board. But, in the end, he served on the Alcan board for less than a year. When Burlingame left the Alcan board, he told me that he wasn't used to being a director of a company where management came to the directors before it had actually made up its own mind. Most CEOs feel that they have to come to the board with their mind made up, leaving the directors with very little option. The directors either agree or they disagree, and if they disagree, they don't do that too often before there's a movement to remove the CEO. I never felt that I was showing weakness when I came to the board with a proposal before making the actual decision. My view at Alcan was that we had this group of directors with great intelligence and experience, and if we got them involved, surely they could help us make a better decision.

So when it came to outside directors, I would choose individuals who would speak up at meetings and not be averse to providing me with advice. I never saw the point of a board that was nothing but a rubber stamp. We had some great board members at Alcan like John Nichol, an outspoken entrepreneur and onetime senator from British Columbia, and Ted Newall, who for many years led DuPont Canada. What I really appreciated was the fact that when there was a real problem with management in the company some of these directors wouldn't hesitate to chip in and show up for work for a time. I can think of the tragic situation that arose at our Mexican subsidiary where the fellow running the business died suddenly at a young age, and one of the directors immediately volunteered to fill in as chief executive on a temporary basis.

While I appreciated being asked to join boards as an outside director, there were some invitations I just wouldn't accept. That was the case for the big Canadian banks. The Royal Bank of Canada had long been one of Alcan's key bankers, and Rowland Frazee, the chairman and a good friend, asked me to join his board. Rowlie couldn't believe it when I said no. When he asked me why, I gave him two reasons. "The first is that I don't look forward to being one of fifty-two." You needed a small stadium to hold that many board members, and nobody could convince me that a board that massive could act in an effective way. "Secondly," I explained, "Alcan always had two major banks, and if I went on the board of one of them it would spoil the relationship with the other bank." Rowlie promised to reduce the size of his board, which I agreed was a step in the right direction but not enough to convince me to join the Royal Bank. Conrad Black has written that he's the only Canadian who has ever turned down a Royal Bank directorship. There's at least one other.

The other board that I greatly enjoyed was the J.P. Morgan International Council, not a board of directors per se, but an advisory group with no corporate responsibilities. Those were the days when J.P. Morgan was a really good bank run by good people. The chairman of the council was George Shultz, the former US secretary of state. There were brilliant individuals on it like Geoffrey Howe, who was a leading minister in Margaret Thatcher's government, and Riley Bechtel, chairman of the family-run construction giant. We would often meet in New York where J.P. Morgan was based but at international locations as well, including China.

J.P. Morgan would plan the meetings very carefully, and they would always have their current and former chief executives – three or four of them – present, and so you would have some of these experienced old-timers of the US financial system sitting at the back of the room listening in. I never quite understood what the bank got out of it, although it presumably helped the bank's top executives understand world economic and political trends. For members of the International Council, like me, the meetings were always exceptionally informative.

It's also through George Shultz that I became a member of the advisory council of the Stanford Institute for International Studies, another group that included a selection of leaders in politics, academia, and business. That group included Helmut Schmidt, the former West German chancellor. I remember sitting beside Herr Schmidt one day in the era before the widespread ban on smoking. Schmidt was simultaneously smoking a cigarette and inhaling snuff. He clearly wasn't getting enough nicotine from the cigarette alone.

I went out on a limb and spent a lot of time, money, and effort fighting for the Canada–US Free Trade Agreement in the late 1980s. Together with Tom d'Aquino of the Business Council on National Issues, we got people like Peter Lougheed, the former Alberta premier, Donald Macdonald, the onetime Liberal finance minister, and various other people involved, and we ran a serious campaign through the Canadian Alliance for Trade and Job Opportunities that had some effect. At the height of the free trade debate, the CBC organized a roundtable discussion at Maison Alcan with various people including *La Presse* columnist Lysiane Gagnon and writer Mordecai Richler, a noted tippler who could be a bit mischievous at times. Being active in the free trade debate, I was there as host. At Alcan, we had a young man who acted as the company's chauffeur and butler. Just before the discussion began at 3 p.m., I said to him, "Around 3:30, bring in a breadbasket with a napkin over it. Instead of putting bread inside, include a tumbler of brandy. Put the basket down in front of Mr Richler without saying a word." At the appropriate time, the young man delivered the breadbasket to Mordecai who was in full flourish, opining on something or other. Mordecai reached out, lifted the napkin and spied the brandy. His face lit up. He was much easier to handle after that.

These advisory councils and other interests, along with the Seagram and Amex boards, took a fair bit of my time so I decided to accept a place on only one other US board, that of American Cyanamid, a fine company that unfortunately no longer exists. It was involved in a wide range of businesses, including agricultural chemicals, fibers, pharmaceuticals, and consumer products. Although the parent company may not have been a household name, its stable of products included well-established brands like Centrum vitamins, Breck shampoo, Old Spice aftershave, and Formica building products. Before accepting the invitation to join the company's board, I consulted Alcan's legal firm in New York. I discovered that American Cyanamid's roots were in Pittsburgh, and its pedigree was very similar to Alcan's. Cyanamid's original backers were established Pittsburgh families, like the Mellons and the Hunts, who also had invested in Alcoa and Alcan. My first American Cyanamid board meeting was just before Christmas, and, as was the company tradition, the December meeting took place in New York City at the 21 Club, which was about as fancy as you could get. When I walked into that meeting with the other directors and members of management, I felt something familiar. It was the same corporate culture as Alcan. There were no party politics, and nobody was trying to stab anybody else in the back. Nobody was trying to crawl over anybody else on the way up.

My presence on the board lasted until 1994 when Cyanamid became the object of an unfriendly takeover bid by American Home Products. The opening price was $95 a share, representing a premium of more than fifty per cent above the stock price at the time. We had some pretty intense board meetings about how to respond, and during one of those encounters a law firm served the Cyanamid directors, including myself, with a class action lawsuit on behalf of the shareholders. We were being sued for not accepting American Home Products' bid of $95. To me, it was another case of the lunatic nature of the American legal system. We hadn't even decided as a board whether to accept or reject the bid, and already we were being sued for not accepting it. It was nuts. The directors went ahead with the meeting to mull over the bid. We decided that the best thing to do as a board was to talk with American Home Products and encourage them to increase their offer to a point where we could work with them rather than against them. We did exactly that and we finally got American Home Products to agree to increase its bid to $101 a share.

At that point, the same law firm brought a second class action suit against us for not getting a price higher than $101! More craziness. As a result of that lawsuit, I was subpoenaed as an outside director to be examined in court. To add to my irritation, they chose a Sunday at 11 a.m. in New Jersey, near Cyanamid's headquarters, for the deposition. I had to leave Manitou at 5 a.m. to drive to Montreal and get on a Cyanamid company plane that had been flown up to take me to the hearing. Once I got there, this prissy American lawyer questioned me for a total of six hours with a court stenographer taking it all down. Finally, he asked me, "On what basis did you reach the conclusion that you could not get more than $101 a share?" Just then, I remembered reading somewhere that no judge likes to substitute his judgment for the judgment of somebody with a boatload of experience. So I answered, "Forty-five years of international business experience has told me that we couldn't get a cent more than $101." Clearly not happy with my response, the lawyer glared at me and said, "OK, that's all." And the hearing was over.

When I flew home to Montreal that evening I knew that this time, at least, I had done my duty as an outside director and served the shareholders well.

11

"Hitting the Right Note"

The Meaning of Pastimes

I've always believed in the importance of balance in life, of the need to make sure that no one part of life dominated everything else. I never could understand how people could work sixteen-hour days for weeks at a time or go into the office every Sunday whether there was a crisis or not. I was never one of those businessmen who thought that being home in time for dinner with the family, going to the symphony, or playing a round of golf somehow meant that I was a less effective C E O. This concept of balance in life was inculcated in me from an early age by my parents, who believed in studying diligently and working hard but also in pursuing pastimes like music or golf or tennis.

As was expected of children in my time, I took piano lessons starting from the age of six from a certain Miss Johnson in her studio on Sherbrooke Street opposite Westmount Park. I wasn't particularly good at practising and didn't seem destined to be another Horowitz, so when I turned twelve I asked my mother to let me quit, and she agreed. Yet I never stopped tinkering with the piano and continued to play popular music, something I still have fun doing almost a lifetime later. In 1947, when I travelled to Europe for the summer, I was determined to do one serious thing while I was abroad. That's how I came to take piano lessons for two months in Paris and learn something about how to play the instrument properly.

I arrived in France with one suit of clothes, one pair of shoes, and a suitcase full of contraband – sugar, coffee, cigarettes, silk stockings – precious items I was told would be worth more than cash in a country still suffering from postwar shortages. The ship landed in Le Havre, and I travelled from there to Paris by train. We had to go through a customs inspection on the train, and, considering my contraband-filled suitcase, I wasn't looking forward to it. I boarded the train and started walking down the corridor looking for a place to sit in one of the separate passenger compartments then common to European trains. I spied one compartment, designed for six passengers, which had just one elderly lady seated alongside a pile of suitcases. This looked like a good place to be when it was time for the customs inspection. I carefully opened the door to test the waters, and the woman looked daggers at me, clearly not pleased at the appearance of a young interloper in her domain. Nevertheless, I judiciously moved one of her suitcases aside, enough so that I could sit down, and put my suitcase strategically amongst hers. A short time later, the French customs officer opened the door with a flourish and looked at all the luggage, then over at the elderly lady and said, "Madame n'a rien à déclarer, n'est-ce pas?" She replied, "Mais non! Rien!" Then the officer looked at me and commented, "Comme les dames sont bizarres," and left. That's how I managed to get to Paris with my contraband undisturbed.

I headed for a boarding house in the Sixteenth Arrondissement where I had made an arrangement to stay, or at least I thought I had. It was located in a grand old residence run by a formerly titled Russian lady with the extraordinary name of Madame Dargouzh-Gonzetti, a tiny woman who must have weighed at most ninety-five pounds. My mother had a friend from Montreal, a Mrs Ryan, who had stayed at this place, and Mrs Ryan had supposedly written a letter of introduction on my behalf. Reflecting what must have been a sharp fall from her perch in the pre-1917 Russian aristocracy, Madame Dargouzh-Gonzetti was perpetually short of cash. Where she got money to feed her fifteen boarders in postwar

Paris, I don't know. I arrived at about six o'clock one evening and rang the doorbell. This frail elderly woman opened the door a crack and immediately said, "Non!" as if I were some unwanted missionary anxious to convert her to an exotic religion. I told her who I was and that I was a friend of Mrs Ryan from Canada, who I thought had arranged for me to stay there. Madame Dargouzh-Gonzetti was adamant. "Non, non. Pas possible! Pas possible!" Starting to panic that I was about to be homeless, I pleaded with her, "Qu'est-ce que je vais faire? Peut-être je peux téléphoner?" She looked at me suspiciously. Then I said, pointing to my valise, "Je dois chercher le numéro." Of course, I had no phone number to look for and nobody to call. I just wanted an excuse to open my suitcase and show her my treasures. I flipped open the bag non-chalantly and pretended to start searching for the phone number. Madame Dargouzh-Gonzetti saw the stash of goodies in the suitcase, and her tone changed remarkably. "Venez avec moi," she said, ushering me into her home. That's how I got a room there. In the end, I gave her practically everything in the suitcase, and she deserved every bit of it!

The summer of 1947 proved to be exceedingly hot. The room next to me was occupied by a Catholic priest who was always dressed in heavy black robes. I'm not sure how he managed to survive in the unrelenting heat, but every afternoon at around four o'clock he would knock on my door and, to keep me out of trouble, ask me to go for a walk in the Bois de Boulogne. These walks proved to be a fabulous immersion course in the French that I had not had enough opportunity to use back in Montreal. There were other interesting people staying in the rooming house, including a young woman who was about thirty years old, a heroine of the war who had smuggled Allied airmen out of France. During the two months I was there, at least four or five English guys dropped in to thank her for getting them to safety.

With my musical education in mind, I asked Madame Dargouzh-Gonzetti if I could rent a piano. She agreed and said that I could put the piano in the salon. The house had a huge front room that was never used and where every surface was covered with sheets as if the occupants had disappeared on a lengthy vacation or simply skipped town. I rented a piano and began practising daily in the otherwise unused room. One morning, I heard Madame Dargouzh-Gonzetti go out the front door and head down the street on some errands. Just then a neighbour yelled at her from a window above, "Madame, Madame, ce piano, ce tap-tap-tap, ce n'est pas joli! C'est pas joli du tout!" After a long pause, Madame Dargouzh-Gonzetti responded, "Quel piano, eh? Quel piano?" She paid no attention to the neighbour and encouraged me to study under a professor at the conservatory. He gave me occasional piano lessons and introduced me to a colleague, a music historian and renowned organist named Norbert Dufourcq.

I called Monsieur Dufourcq and asked him if I could study music history with him. He said he would mull it over and asked me to meet him at nine o'clock at night at Notre Dame Cathedral, the magnificent church on Ile de la Cité. Arriving at the appointed time, I opened the door and discovered that the inside of the church was pitch black. Feeling my way along a wall, I eventually discerned a single light bulb casting a yellow glow way up in the organ loft. It was the only light in the whole building. I climbed the stairs into the loft, and there was Monsieur Dufourcq playing Bach, energetically going at the organ with his feet and hands. He nodded at me to turn the pages, which I did for half an hour as he played this beautiful organ music in an absolutely empty church, the perspiration dripping off his face in the oppressive summer heat. I'll never forget that sight.

I went once a week to each of my music teachers that summer. It proved to be simultaneously the apex and the end of my formal musical training because once I went home to Montreal I never took another piano lesson. Yet, in the decades that followed, I never stopped fiddling around with the piano. I would play the piano at parties as a student, not brilliantly but well enough for people to sing along with. Even now, I like to sit down after dinner and play for fifteen minutes or so. My repertoire consists of what I call cocktail music for old ladies. That's the kind of music I prefer, old favourites like *Over the Rainbow* and *Stardust*. My first reaction whenever I enter a new home is to look for the piano because, for me, a house is not a home without a piano. I have one at the Lac Manitou house and another at my apartment in Montreal. I used to have a piano at Maison Alcan, in the reception room next to the Atholstan House boardroom. My one regret about my house in Georgia is that I don't have a piano there yet.

While I also enjoy listening to music, I don't often sit at home to the sounds of a symphony recording. I do go to the Montreal Symphony concerts and enjoy being there. I have been a longtime supporter and board member of the McGill Chamber Orchestra, but I'm not what you might call a musical aficionado. I have a theory about appreciating music. I believe that it is impossible to enjoy music you don't know, that you're not familiar with. The bottom line is that it's really hard to enjoy a piece when you're hearing it for the first time. That's because when you know a piece you sense the sound that is going to be played before it's actually played, and if the sound that's played meshes smoothly and completely with what you're sensing, you become fulfilled. If you aren't able to sense the next tone that will be struck, you're not able to match it up.

I love Dixieland music, and I love good jazz. Above all, I love a good piano player who doesn't hit too many notes. And I even love a few who do, like Oliver Jones and the late Oscar Peterson. When I celebrated my eightieth birthday a few years back, my dear friend Herbie Black threw a lovely party for me at his home in Westmount, with Oliver Jones providing the entertainment. Talk about a dream gift! My longtime interest in jazz prompted me to have Alcan sign up as one of the first corporate sponsors of the Montreal International Jazz Festival, which has become a well-loved institution in the city and a cornerstone of its summer festival scene.

I didn't have to go beyond Alcan to find one of the best jazz piano players I've heard anywhere. Patrick Rich was above all a first-class manager, but he has real talent as a musician as well, and, strangely enough, that came to the fore when we were on a business trip together in the 1980s. We were working to expand Alcan's business and heard of a German steel company that was interested in investing in aluminum. One Thursday morning, we called the firm and asked to see them at their headquarters close to the Dutch border. When they responded that they could see us the next day, we jumped on a K L M flight that night from Montreal to Amsterdam, dressed in our business suits and carrying nothing but our briefcases. We rented a car and drove to Germany to see them. Our plan was to get back to Amsterdam later that day in time to catch the 5 p.m. flight back to Montreal and be home for the weekend. But, sure enough, we missed the flight. Stranded in Amsterdam, we decided to stay over and take a plane home on Saturday. We booked a room at a downtown hotel, took a shower, got back in our business suits, and headed down to the hotel bar.

While sitting there, I asked the bartender whether there was a place in Amsterdam that played Latin American jazz, which I knew was Patrick's specialty. The bartender reached down under the bar and handed me a thick directory with a long list of jazz clubs. I found a page that listed Latin American clubs, put my finger on a random spot on the page, and took down the address. When we gave the address to our taxi driver, he responded straightaway, "I'm not allowed to drive you there. I'll take you as far as I can, but you'll have to walk the rest of the way." Arriving at the club in the middle of Amsterdam's red light district, I pushed open the door and was engulfed by a strong smell of marijuana. I could hear a small band playing Latin American jazz at the far end of the room. We took off our ties, ordered a couple of beers, and sat down next to a fortyish guy with a beard and who was dressed in denim decorated with lots of flowers – shades of San Francisco in 1968.

As the band came to the end of its set, the piano player exclaimed, "Pat! Is that you, Pat?" Patrick Rich turned to me and explained, "You won't believe this, but I used to play in New York with this guy." Patrick took off his suit jacket, stepped on stage, and sat down at the piano at which point the guy with the beard said, "Pat? Well, I know all the jazz pianists, but I don't know any Pat. Where does he play?" I responded, "He doesn't. He's an amateur." The guy pressed on, "If he doesn't play, what does he do for a living?" I responded in deadpan, "He's the president of a multinational company." Those were the days when it wasn't exactly popular to be a multinational executive, particularly in a jazz bar in inner-city Amsterdam. The guy took a long look at me and said, "Hey man, what are you on?" Patrick and I spent the next four or five hours in that seedy bar having the time of our lives. The music was fantastic, and Patrick played half of the sets himself. I still tell him that was the best business trip I ever had.

I always thought that as far as Alcan was concerned our support for music should not simply be one of providing financial assistance for organizations like the Montreal Symphony or the Jazz Festival. Music should be integrated into company activities. So when we moved to Maison Alcan, I encouraged the holding of lunchtime musical events in the building's atrium so as to benefit headquarters employees and members of the public. Since Alcan was bought by Rio Tinto, unfortunately that approach has been abandoned. The front doors are shut to the public and the atrium that was once a restful public space for art and music is just another office building lobby. Now that Rio Tinto has sold the building and announced that Alcan will be moving to new rented quarters in the Deloitte Tower, it is my hope that the new owners of Maison Alcan will revitalize the complex and reintegrate it into Montreal's social and cultural life.

My first big-time experience with sponsorship came in 1967 when I helped convince Alcan to sponsor what was then the biggest golfing event in the world, the Alcan Golfer of the Year Championship. Our goal was to get Alcan's name and brand distinguished from Alcoa's, and we figured that frequent mention of the Alcan name in the world's press would be an effective way to do so. The championship offered the biggest prize money in golf at the time, $40,000 for first prize and $25,000 for second prize, attracting the best golfers in the world. The first event was held at the Royal & Ancient Club at St Andrews in Scotland, with Gay Brewer the winner. Brewer won again the next year at Royal Birkdale in England, followed by Billy Casper in 1969 when the championship was held in Portland, Oregon. Bruce Devlin won the last one in 1970 at Portmarnock in Ireland.

There never was a fifth year because the bosses of professional golf organized the schedule so that the only date available for Alcan's tournament in 1971 was baseball's World Series week, which put the event in an impossibly uncompetitive situation. It turned out that Mark McCormack of IMG, the big sports management company, was no friend of Alcan and helped sink the tournament. He was angry that we didn't use him as a promoter and didn't like the fact that we hadn't provided for sponsor's exemptions. We had invested big money in Alcan Golfer of the Year, but it was money well spent since it attracted lots of ink and helped establish Alcan as an international brand.

For me, golf was always a lot more than a corporate sponsorship tool. It's been part of my life since I was a boy, and I've seen the sport grow in its geographic range and its appeal spread to a much broader public. I've played golf on every continent, in Iceland at the world's northernmost golf course, and in Invercargill, New Zealand, what may be the globe's southernmost golf course. And, I've played in every sort of weather. I can still remember a game with the chairman of the Hyundai conglomerate in Korea. It was early December, and there had been a dusting of snow overnight so members of the chairman's entourage rushed around sweeping snow off every fairway where the chairman's ball usually landed. Golf was important to me for its restorative powers as well. When I used to travel to Australia on business, it would take thirty-two hours to get from my house in Montreal to the airport in Sydney. I would arrive in Sydney at 7 a.m., and John Clarkson, Alcan's Area Manager in the region, would pick me up and drive me directly to the golf course. We would play eighteen holes, and at four o'clock he would deliver me back to the hotel where I'd hit the sack and sleep until eight the next morning. That's how I got over the long trip. The man who used to run Rio Tinto in the 1970s was Sir Val Duncan, an inveterate traveler. I once asked him what he did when he arrived home in London after a long airplane trip.

He responded, "I always do the same thing. I go to the foot of my garden, I lie down on the ground, and I have a good sleep. My theory is that after you've been in the air for a long time, get as close to the ground as you can." My equivalent of doing that was to play golf after a long trip. That got me close to the ground.

For some, golf has an almost religious attraction, which might be one way of explaining a special devotion to the sport I experienced in Ireland. In the late 1970s, Alcan was embarking on a massive project on the Emerald Isle, the Aughinish alumina refinery. I flew to Ireland in the Alcan plane to attend the sod-turning ceremony and landed at around 7 p.m. Irish time, which was still 2 p.m. back in Montreal. I arrived in time for a big dinner that included the local Roman Catholic bishop and all the other big wigs who were going to be at the ceremony. The entertainment included guitars and an Irish balladeer, with everybody singing and weeping. I finally got to bed at 4 a.m., which was still only 11 p.m. my time. My room was a cavernous affair in Dromoland Castle, an historic pile that had been turned into a hotel. At 7 a.m., after just three hours of sleep, my phone rang. I picked it up and this lilting Irish voice said, "Mr Culver, my name is Jim Newman. I'm the local priest here and I understand that you like to play golf. If you get out of bed and are downstairs in twenty minutes, I'll take you to Ballybunion, and we can have a round of golf and still be back in time for the sod turning at three." Not wanting to miss the opportunity to play golf on one of the world's legendary courses, I rushed downstairs and the priest picked me up in a flivver of a car. We headed first to the presbytery where Father Jim picked up his own clubs and a golf bag belonging to another priest, a tiny bag with a lot of assorted clubs sticking out of it, that he had kindly lent to me.

It was not until I got to the first tee at Ballybunion and took the cover off one of the clubs that I could see it was a handmade Smith driver costing about $300 in those days. "Your colleague has a pretty nice club here," I commented. "Ah," Father Jim responded, "It's a gift from a parishioner." We played golf in the wind and the rain on that challenging but breathtaking course. Jim shot a seventy-three. As we were driving to the sod turning after our round of golf, I said, "By the way, your colleague whose clubs I used, does he play golf as well as you do?" Jim responded, "Oh, he's much better than I am. I never beat him." "How old is he?" I asked. "Oh, he'd be in his 60s," Father Jim replied. I told him I was pretty impressed. As I got up on the dais for the sod-turning ceremony, I met the bishop, a huge man who was probably six-foot-six tall and weighed about 280 pounds. He sported a big red sash, a red skull-cap, and an equally red face. When there was a pause in the ceremony, I turned to him and said, "I must say I'm pretty impressed with the golfing ability of your priests around here." The bishop took a quick look around to see whether anybody was listening, leaned over, and whispered to me, "It's all they bloody well do!"

I started playing golf at the Murray Bay Golf Club in Pointe-au-Pic when I was nine years old. My brother Bronson and I used to run down the hill from our summer house and cross the railway tracks to the club. It was an eighteen-hole course, and if it was a rainy day and nobody was around we would play the course three times in one day, a total of fifty-four holes. I loved the game from the start, and I always found it to be an excellent test of mental and physical self-control. I was fortunate to have been born with good hand-to-eye coordination, which meant that I always had a certain skill in ball games like squash, tennis, and golf. Occasionally for a real treat, my father would take us to the course at the Manoir Richelieu. He was a pretty good golfer, but, like me, he hit from the top all the time.

My mother was an excellent golfer and loved the game. In 1969, the year after my father died, Fern was invited by one of her friends in the travel business to tour Hawaii on an all-expense-paid trip. They were three ladies of a certain age, of whom Fern was the only golfer. One of their stops was at my favourite hotel, the Mauna Kea Beach Hotel on the Big Island, where I ended up going with Mary every winter for thirty-three years. As you arrive at the property, which I consider to be the most romantic resort in the world, there's a long drive through this beautiful golf course to get to the hotel. My mother was dying to play golf, and as soon as she got to the hotel she decided to book a golf lesson. She took it for granted that some nice man would be the golf pro. Fern was an outspoken woman but no feminist. She didn't like women doing what she called "men's work," and so imagine her horror when she discovered that the pro at Mauna Kea was Jackie Pung, one of the early women to make a name for herself on the golf circuit. Although Jackie was a large Hawaiian lady and quite imposing, it didn't stop Fern from attempting to lord over her, boasting that she had taken lessons from the likes of Tommy Armour and Sam Snead, and telling her that being a golf pro was really a man's job.

Jackie Pung took it all in stride. "Well, Mrs Culver, why don't you show me how you hit the ball?" My mother did what she always did. She hit the ball 105 yards down the middle of the fairway with every subsequent shot identical to the previous one. Jackie Pung was courteous and asked, "Mrs Culver, what don't you like about your swing?" My mother replied, "The ball doesn't go far enough! That's what I don't like." Jackie stepped up to her and said, "Now, Mrs Culver, you've played a lot of golf in your life. You know a lot about the game. I don't have to tell you that if you want to hit the ball farther you've got to clear your left side. That's how you get the ball away. Now, I'll tell you something that those fancy pros never told you. There's only one way for you and me to clear the left side, and that is to push your left breast out of the way and then swing. Push it under your arm and then swing." My mother always said that was the best damned golf lesson she ever had!

When I was a boy, my parents belonged to the Royal Montreal Golf Club, or Dixie as it was popularly known, but decided to switch to the Mount Bruno Golf Club sometime during the Second World War. Bruno, as we call it, is a nice club with no start times and fewer people, which means there is less pressure. Royal Montreal had been founded as an initiative of the Bank of Montreal many years earlier. The general manager of the Royal Bank, the Bank of Montreal's crosstown rival, was determined not to be outdone and decided to back a new golf course at Mount Bruno, on the South Shore of the St Lawrence River. He chose 1918 as the starting date, but in the end he had to deal with the recession of

1919–20, which really saved the course from itself. If there hadn't been that recession, Mount Bruno would have gone ahead with its original plan for a huge stone, castle-like clubhouse. Instead, they decided to live with their so-called "temporary" Tudor-style clubhouse, which is still there today and, in the opinion of many people, is one of the nicest clubhouses anywhere because of its simplicity. The course itself was designed by Willy Park Jr, a famous golf architect from Scotland who designed many great golf courses in North America. And even though the area has been built up considerably with suburban development, when you're playing you see nothing but the golf course. It's a lovely place, and when I'm up on the hill on a summer's evening I wonder why I'm not there every night.

I was president of Bruno in 1969–70, at the tender age of 45. I sometimes remind the members that today there aren't many golf clubs still serving meals to someone who was president more than forty years ago. It was a bit of a stretch for me to take on the role since I was travelling a lot for Alcan, prompting some wags to call me Bruno's absentee president. Yet I managed to accomplish a few things in my tenure of which I am still proud. I started the club's first practice fairway, and, most importantly, I brought in its first francophone members, a move that did not get the unanimous backing of some of the old-line anglo members. Today, I would say that Bruno is 40 per cent francophone, 40 per cent anglophone, and 20 per cent that special Montreal category, allophone. I figured that if we wanted Mount Bruno to be the best golf club in Montreal, it had to reflect the best of Montreal. What's interesting is that I now play more golf than ever before. In the past three years, I have played twice as much as I used to.

Golf may be a great business tool, but in Canada fishing, and in particular salmon fishing, is when many of the important decisions and relationships are made. It's when business people and politicians can truly relax, get to know each other, and discuss important issues without the interruptions of the outside world. No meetings, no email, often no telephone, just long days in hip waders contemplating the beauty of a salmon stream and hoping for one to bite, followed by cool evenings by the fire with good food, drink, and companionship.

What you need above all to be a good fisherman is a love of solitude and lots of patience. I always remind people that it's called fishing not catching. I've been on weeklong fishing trips during which I didn't see a single fish. John Grimston, the seventh Earl of Verulam, a British M P, wartime R A F pilot, and chairman of Delta Metals, one of Alcan's most loyal British customers, was also the best fisherman I ever met. His family owned a large estate in Scotland that boasted great salmon rivers, and he frequently came to Canada to fish as a guest of Alcan. Lord Verulam once told me that even if you go to the best rivers in the world at the right time and under the right conditions, it still takes an average of five hours of casting to catch a single fish. There are some people who just aren't cut out to spend five hours without a tug on the line.

One thing that many fishermen do during those five hours of anticipation and frustration is to come up with all sorts of reasons why they're not catching anything. Stephen Leacock, the great humourist, had a pond outside his house in Orillia, Ontario. There wasn't a single fish in it, but he used to ask trout fishermen he knew to bring along their tackle and try their luck in the pond. When they came back with nothing after several hours, they always had a reason: the water temperature was wrong, or the moon was wrong, or some other far-fetched excuse. Leacock once made the mistake of inviting a guy who he thought was an experienced fisherman but really wasn't one. After spending a frustrating half hour at the pond, the would-be fisherman came back empty handed and said simply, "There are no damned fish in that pond!"

To me, the excitement is when the fish makes a pass at the fly but doesn't take it the first time. You know there's a fish that's interested, and the fun is how to get him hooked. Once I've landed him, all I want to do is safely release him back into the water in good shape. I love fishing, but I don't like dealing with dead fish and cooking and eating them. I'd rather release them. I like eating fish, but somehow I don't get any kick out of killing a fish that I've caught.

The fishing camp closest to my heart remains the Sainte-Marguerite Salmon Club, located just north of Tadoussac on Quebec's Sainte-Marguerite River, a tributary of the Saguenay. I've been a member there since 1957, when my late father-in-law, Rip Powell, owned it. In the early part of the nineteenth century, when the Hudson Bay Co. had a trading post at Tadoussac, English army and naval officers would canoe up to the mouth of the Sainte-Marguerite to fish for the abundant salmon. The area around the camp was first logged by the Price brothers, who later established the pulp and paper company that carried the family name, and it was a Price who first obtained a lease from the government for salmon privileges along the river. At the club there's still a photograph of King Edward VII, when he was Prince of Wales, being carried on the back of a Price family member across the mouth of the Sainte-Marguerite River during the prince's visit to Canada in 1860. A clubhouse was built in 1872 and is still in use.

The club was formally established by a group of Americans in the 1880s. They were mostly men of letters, poets, and writers who came from northern New York State, from towns like Utica, Oswego, and Rochester, as well as from Philadelphia and New York City. They would leave home in the middle of June, travel down the St Lawrence River by boat, stay at the camp for two months, and then head home. The fishing log for a single summer would read something like 1,000 salmon and 12,000 trout taken. Truly amazing when you think that today we release virtually every fish that we catch. The official catch limit now is one fish per rod per day, and the only thing you can keep is a grilse, which is a teenage salmon that's too young to breed. Otherwise all of the salmon go back into the river.

The camp was a particular favourite of Walter Brackett, a well-known Boston painter who specialized in still lifes of salmon and trout. Here's an account from the *Quebec Chronicle* newspaper of July 1892 on activities at the camp that summer: "Mr Walter Brackett, the fish painter of Boston, and his family are whipping their pools on the Sainte-Marguerite and the waters of the Sainte-Marguerite Fishing Club, on the same stream being fished by Messrs. Williams, Mitchell and Barney of New York and Mr Lyons of Oswego. Mr Blanchard of Boston has fished the same river for several days and killed but two fish, one of 37 pounds and the other but little over 11." Some of those New Yorkers were original club members and have left their names on the fish pools that are still regularly used by anglers, but I confess to some satisfaction that the best pool on the whole river is known as the Culver Pool.

In the early part of the twentieth century, people went by boat overnight from Montreal to Tadoussac. Then they were driven about twelve miles along a dirt road. The car would stop by the side of the river, and the men, who in those days travelled in suits and fedoras, would scamper down the banks of the river and into canoes. Then they canoed down the river and over the rapids and ended up at the camp. By the time you finally got there, you really felt like you were far away from everything. Today you can drive right to the camp although it still maintains its original ambience, including some of the original wood cottages with their steep roofs and white and green trim.

Rip Powell bought the whole camp for next to nothing from its American owners during the Second World War and used it mainly for business. In the 1970s, he decided to sell the camp to Alcan, which had long used it to entertain clients and friends of the company. Mr Powell told me he wanted to sell the camp for what he considered to be a fair price and asked me to act as the intermediary. He had visions of it being worth around $1 million, but Nat Davis, Alcan's CEO, wasn't about to bite, if you'll pardon the expression. As the frugal grandson of a Protestant minister, Nat had spent years squirming when he saw the expense accounts of the Alcan people who used to take customers up to the camp. Mr Powell may have owned the fishing camp, but Alcan had long paid the expenses, and Nat's view was that Alcan had already paid for the Sainte-Marguerite facility many times over. He hired Royal Trust to put a valuation on the camp and they came up with a price of $35,000. When I told Mr Powell, he looked at me and said, "Whose side are you on anyway?" In the end, Alcan got its way on price. The club was always a draw for our clients and partners, particularly with the Europeans from Alusuisse and Pechiney after Alcan purchased both companies. It now belongs to Rio Tinto, but it continues to be run pretty much as it was in the past. Membership in the club is cheap but it costs about $1,500 per person per day to fish there.

Lots of important relationships were developed at the camp and plenty of Canadian political history was decided there. C.D. Howe, Canada's Minister of Everything during the Second World War and a man whom I admired tremendously, would be a regular visitor. He would travel with Mr Powell and a few of their buddies for a week of fishing. In contrast, we only go for a few days at a time now. Premier Maurice Duplessis was also a frequent guest. Over the years, my guests at the club have included Malcolm Fraser, the former Australian prime minister, David Johnston, our current governor general, Alastair Gillespie, a onetime federal cabinet minister, Paul Volcker, onetime head of the US Federal Reserve, and John Smale, chairman of Procter & Gamble.

In the summer of 1974, just after the federal election that saw Pierre Trudeau's Liberals win a majority after a campaign focused on its opposition to wage and price controls, Finance Minister John Turner and Simon Reisman, his deputy minister, came to the club at my invitation. Turner was actually a bit disappointed at the election result, having hoped that Trudeau would lose, allowing him to take over leadership of the Liberal Party. It was an ambition that Turner would have to wait another decade to achieve, and by that time it proved to be a poisoned chalice. When Turner and Reisman arrived at the fishing camp, I introduced John to the fishing guide I had chosen for him, Normand Dufour, from one of the local families whose members had worked at the camp for generations. John was still in his handshaking mode from the election campaign and greeted Normand, an engaging fellow in his early thirties. Launching into politician small talk, John asked Normand what he did in the off-season. Normand responded that he had been on *chômage* the previous winter, collecting unemployment insurance. "I guess jobs are hard to find around here in the winter," John responded sympathetically. No, said Normand, getting work wasn't really a problem because he was a licensed Hydro-Québec lineman. When John then wondered why he had been on *chômage*, Normand responded that he was building a house and it was better to be on *chômage* than at work, especially when Mr Stanfield had threatened to limit his salary to $5.75 an hour if he got elected rather than the $6.50 an hour that Normand had been counting on. "That was not very smart of Mr Stanfield," Normand commented. When John protested that inflation was an important issue that somehow needed to be addressed, Normand wasn't convinced. "Not when you live here in the country. I grow my own food. I make my own jam. I don't feel any inflation here. I feel inflation when my salary is limited to $5.75 an hour instead of $6.50. That's when I feel inflation."

John Turner turned to me and said with a twinkle in his eye, "You know, you've got to get out into the countryside to really learn the facts." A year later, John quit the cabinet and returned to private life after refusing in his 1975 budget to impose wage and price controls. Donald Macdonald succeeded him in the finance portfolio and in October 1975 introduced the kind of wage and price controls that the Liberals had campaigned against just a year earlier. Who knows? Maybe that encounter with Normand Dufour at the club had a role in determining John's views.

For many years, access to Sainte Marguerite was difficult, but in the early 1960s, against Mr Powell's wishes, the Quebec government built a road from Tadoussac to Chicoutimi, parallel to the river. That road greatly disturbed the riverbanks, leading to a deterioration of many fish pools, which got filled in with gravel and silt. Over time, the situation has improved, but nevertheless considerable damage was done. At the same time, pressure began to mount from the locals who resented being barred from fishing in what they considered their own backyard by private clubs like the Sainte-Marguerite. The Parti Québécois fed the movement for *déclubbage*, arguing that private fishing clubs were dominated by *les anglais* and wealthy Americans at the expense of ordinary Quebecers.

Poaching became a big problem. We had guards on the river, but they couldn't protect the whole length of it. Sometime in the mid-1960s we caught a guy poaching. We decided to make an example of him and took him to court, where he was fined $500, a large amount of money in those days. Fast forward about ten years or so and the Parti Québécois under René Lévesque gets elected. Who should turn up in his cabinet as minister responsible for fisheries but that very same poacher! Part of the P Q's platform was to end the supposed privileges of the province's private fishing clubs. So, the very first *zone d'exploitation contrôlée*, or Z E C, a form of citizen-controlled wildlife area, was on the Sainte-Marguerite River, making part of the river accessible to the public. Call it bad luck or sweet revenge, but, because the Sainte-Marguerite Club had actually owned the riparian rights on several miles of the river since the nineteenth century, the club was one of the few private clubs to survive, although we lost exclusivity on much of the river.

Despite the pressure from additional fishermen that the Z E C brought, the river is now well managed and poaching has all but disappeared. One big advantage of the Z E C system is that the public began to understand the need to protect fish stocks. Part of the river still belongs to the club. There are two branches of the river, the northwest and the northeast. The northwest branch is the one with the road alongside it, which means that it has been badly disturbed. It's no longer the salmon river it used to be, although there are still fish that do go up there. But on the northeast branch there's no road, and four miles up the river there's a waterfall, which the salmon historically couldn't get past. During the 1970s, when I was active in the club, we decided to build a fish ladder up that waterfall, knowing that once the salmon could get up those falls, there was a twelve-mile stretch of wilderness river with great fishing potential. Beyond that, there was an even bigger waterfall, which the salmon would never get past. Two experts, one Canadian and the other from Norway, told me that they could build us a fish ladder for $35,000 that would solve the problem. That proved to be unrealistic, to say the least. It ended up costing us $469,000, or more than ten times as much, but even once this gold-plated ladder was in place, the fish couldn't be convinced to enter into it.

We spent a lot of time and money trying to solve the problem, but nothing worked. The club finally asked the Quebec government to recommend someone who could help us. One day when I was at the camp, a young man knocked at the door, a bearded, intellectual-looking fellow who was probably in his early twenties. Introducing himself as Marc Valentine, he said that he was studying biology at Laval University and knew we were having a problem with the fish ladder but was convinced that he could solve it. When I asked him how he was going to accomplish that feat, he responded that he planned to pitch a tent and live at the mouth of the ladder until he figured out a way to get the fish to swim into it. Sure enough, Valentine spent two summers at the waterfall and painstakingly kept changing the configuration of the ladder until the flow of water was such that the salmon finally found their way into it. It worked, and that twelve-mile stretch of untouched river has turned into a remarkable salmon stream. If you visit that waterfall today, you'll see Marc Valentine's name on the fish ladder to honour his accomplishment. Eventually, the Quebec government bought the fish ladder from Alcan so we now share the fishing rights above the falls with the public. The public has the right to fish on Sundays, and we have the exclusive right to that stretch of water the rest of the week. Membership of the fishing club is still made up largely of current and former employees of Rio Tinto Alcan. I still get an invitation to the club's annual meeting at Maison Alcan.

While I adore the Sainte-Marguerite River, it doesn't compare with the Grand Cascapedia River in the Gaspésie on the border of Quebec and New Brunswick. It is probably the best Atlantic salmon river of them all, with lots of big fish and a history dating back to the 1860s. For many years Izaak and Dorothy Killam owned what was called Middle Camp on the Grand Cascapedia and would travel down from Montreal in their private rail car, in the same way the super-rich use executive jets today. At one point, probably in the 1950s, Dorothy Killam invited my mother down to Middle Camp for some salmon fishing. They were great friends, but Dorothy also asked a boyfriend from New York to come along. So there were Dorothy and her beau, with Fern supposedly acting as the chaperone. This was not unusual for Mrs Killam, who travelled the world socializing while her husband kept on working. Though it was probably all pretty innocent, there's no denying that Mrs Killam enjoyed the company of good-looking men. At one time she wanted to buy the Brooklyn Dodgers. Fern used to say it was because she liked the sight of all those young men in tight pants! All went well at the fishing camp until one evening the boyfriend started dancing with Fern instead of with Dorothy, who was not amused. The next morning, my mother found herself deposited at the railway depot at Matapedia to be sent back to Montreal.

The train pulled up to the station with the Killams' private car attached. Fern climbed aboard the car holding her ticket reading "Mrs Killam." As the train started off, the conductor looked at the ticket and said to my mother, "Mrs Killam, I've never seen you looking so fine." To which my mother replied, "You're damned right you haven't!"

12

"Just Another Graduation"

Life after Alcan

I never made it to sixty-five at Alcan, stepping down six months before I hit the magic number in 1989. There was nothing mysterious about my action. I had joined Alcan on 1 July 1949, and I had become C E O on 1 July 1979, so I decided that 1 July 1989 would be an appropriate date to leave after forty years with the company. It just seemed like the right thing to do. Yet I don't like the term retirement and still use it as little as possible more than twenty years later. There's a finality about "retirement," an indication of withdrawal from active life that I find inaccurate and a bit depressing. I prefer to call this kind of transition "graduation," which indicates both an ending and a new beginning.

I once spoke to the graduating class of my alma mater, Selwyn House, and told the group of seventeen-year-old boys the following. "You guys are sitting there enthusiastic as you can be, looking forward to the next step, and nothing seems to you to be more interesting than what is going to happen next. That kind of enthusiasm is something you want to hold on to all your life. While you are full of enthusiasm now, you don't actually have many options. You have finished high school, and next most of you will graduate from university, still full of enthusiasm, but actually with few options about where you're going to work and what you are going to do with your lives. What happens when you get to sixty-five is that you will have tons of options but little enthusiasm. So the trick is to maintain today's enthusiasm throughout your life." And that's why I hate talking about retirement. I consider it to be just another graduation in the flow of a life.

I was convinced that after ten years of being C E O of a large public company, I should make a total break with Alcan, including leaving the board. The custom at most companies was that a departing C E O remained as a director after stepping down, but I figured this would not be good for the company or for my successor, David Morton. My point was proven at the very first Alcan board meeting after my departure, when the directors approved a form of poison pill that I could never have agreed to. I had an inherent distrust of any move like a poison pill that was designed to hinder competition or halt a takeover. I still feel that it should be possible to deal with these kinds of eventualities in a satisfactory way without the help of a poison pill, which is designed to give the company more time to defend itself. If I had remained as a member of the Alcan board, I would have had to sit there quietly and let the other directors pass the poison pill. Otherwise, I would have undermined the work of my successor just as he was starting.

I had another reason for making the break as complete as possible. I wanted to begin a new career as an investment banker. I had been watching the way that Canada's commercial banks had started to take over the investment banks. Taking lessons from my father's career as an investment banker and having learned from that master of investment banking, I.W. Killam, it seemed evident to me that these takeovers would be a bust. I knew all about the radical differences between the two types of banks, and, to my mind, these corporate marriages were doomed to failure. Yet despite my predictions, the mergers appeared to succeed. What I had missed is that what we were witnessing, in the merger of Canada's chartered banks and the country's leading investment dealers, was a massive reverse takeover.

The investment banks had taken over the commercial banks and, in so doing, had got access to depositors' money, a huge boon to the investment banks because bigger balance sheets allow for bigger deals. From the viewpoint of the commercial banks, the mergers had a special appeal to their top executives. Traditionally, management of the chartered banks had not been paid anything close to what the management of the investment banks earned. In the old days, I can remember when the head of the Royal Bank of Canada was paid something like $25,000 a year. The bank provided him with a big house and a chauffeur and he belonged to lots of clubs, but his paycheque wasn't very big. With the takeover wave of the 1980s, the top brass at Canada's leading banks figured that if they had an investment bank as a subsidiary they'd have to earn more than the management of the investment bank. And that's the way it has turned out.

Convinced initially that these investment house takeovers would ultimately fail, I was anxious to do something I had never done before, which was to start a business from scratch, a traditional investment bank. It was admittedly an increasingly quaint idea, an investment bank that would be owned only by its partners, but I saw nothing wrong with that formula, which put the risk and the reward where it should be, with the partners. With this idea in mind, on 1 July 1989, I walked out of Maison Alcan along with my assistant Janice Darrah, crossed Sherbrooke Street, and hung up my shingle on the ground floor of a three-storey greystone house on Drummond Street that had been converted into offices. The house was actually quite familiar to me. I used to play there as a boy when it was the home of a pediatrician whose son was a friend of mine at Selwyn House.

I brought in my youngest son Mark and a young Danish friend of his named David Kauffmann, and together we formed Culver & Co. Investments, which I conceived of as a small, independent investment bank owned only by its partners. In my forty-year career, I had never been an entrepreneur and had never started anything. Any enterprise I had been involved with was already up and running when I got there. I had never been a financial man, but I had seen how lucrative the investment banking business could be and thought I'd give it a try.

To be honest, I had no idea where to start. As it turned out, I didn't get very far into running Culver & Co. before happenstance once again prompted me to change direction. Within weeks of leaving Alcan, I was in Philadelphia for a meeting. I ran into the street to hail a cab and head to the airport, when another man jumped into the same cab from the other side. It turned out to be Jim Wolfensohn, the Australian-born investment banker whom I had known for some time and was later to become head of the World Bank. He asked me what I was doing now that I had left Alcan and I told him of my plans. After listening for a bit, Jim said, "Why don't you start something in Canada like A E A down here?" I had heard of A E A Investors, which had been founded in 1968 by the Rockefeller, Mellon, and Harriman family interests and S.G. Warburg & Co. In the 1980s, A E A began to raise money from high net-worth individuals and pension funds for investments in leveraged buyouts and midsized companies in an early form of the private equity business. I was intrigued by the idea.

A few weeks later in New York, I ran into Harold Tanner, who had given financial advice to Alcan when he was at Salomon Brothers. Harold asked me what I was doing, and when I went into my description of Culver & Co. he too said, "Why don't you start something like A E A in Canada?" Somebody was trying to send me a message. Finally, I got a call from Dick Schmeelk, a former Salomon Brothers bond dealer who was known in New York as "Mr Canada" because of his involvement with so many Canadian corporate and government deals over the years. Dick said that he and some of his younger colleagues were thinking of starting an A E A-type of business in the US and Canada and asked me whether I would be interested in joining them. Clearly, all three incidents were pointing me in the same direction. The upshot is that I never got started in the investment banking business. I went into private equity instead.

Dick and I cofounded C A I Capital in 1990 with the aim of specializing in investments in Canada and the United States. C A I stands for Canadian American Investors. Our goal was to invest in midsized companies; firms that we felt could be grown and brought to an I P O stage or other kind of sale. At the time, inflation was the order of the day and you could borrow money at almost zero real interest rates. The private equity business was making a lot of money by highly leveraging their deals. They were putting in very little money and making a lot in return. However, we decided that we wanted C A I to last for a long time, much beyond the personal involvement of Dick Schmeelk and myself. We felt that over a long period of time, deflation was going to end up being a bigger problem than inflation so we determined that C A I would make only modest use of credit. I'll admit that this approach didn't work very well for us financially in C A I's Fund I, but it worked a little better in Fund II, and it has worked well in Fund III and Fund IV. We began Fund I in 1990 by raising about $185 million. Our lead investor for that fund and for the subsequent three funds was British Columbia Investment Management Corp., the provincial government's investment manager. The minimum investment for the fund was set at $500,000.

Raising money for that first fund ended up being more difficult than we anticipated. We went around to big pension funds and high-worth individuals in Canada and the US with cap in hand. I had a Rolodex full of excellent contacts, but they were mainly associated with the aluminum industry, and I soon realized that this was a lot different than selling aluminum ingot. Once outside the industry, people looked at me differently. I went to a lot of meetings and got a lot of, "I'll think about it and call you back" from people I never heard from again. I had to learn how to hear *No* in every language there is. It was not much fun. At the start, C A I included five senior people: myself, Dick Schmeelk, plus three somewhat younger guys with whom Dick had previously worked or invested. Added to that core group were my son Mark and his friend David Kauffmann. Today C A I has twenty-two people with offices in Montreal, New York, Toronto, and Vancouver and investments in companies on both sides of the border.

I've never been much of a fan of the kind of private equity deal where you take a tired old company with lots of excess weight, slim it down and turn it into a slender, profitable entity that you sell a short time later for a fortune. You can take any enterprise and slash costs, provided that you're not going to own it for very long. A wise man once said something to me that I still remember. "Downsizing may ensure survival, but it will not ensure success." This kind of private equity firm takes a company that is a little fatter than it needs to be at the moment, slashes costs, and then sells it. By that point, the buyer usually hasn't bought anything that's worth much. We didn't do those kinds of deals at CAI. We were lucky enough to acquire businesses that were genuinely growing.

Looking for investment opportunities was a challenge, but it was a process that I found more rewarding than seeking out money for each fund. I had a different way of approaching it than my partners who would go to banks and other institutions and ask them to bring us deals. My view was that we should back people rather than do deals that came to us wrapped up in some elaborate "sales book," which usually meant that those deals had already been pretty well shopped around to everybody else already. The sales book is made up of a lot of figures that don't make much sense to me anyway. At Alcan, I used to say to people, "Don't give me a plan that's all numbers. Give me words. If the words are right, the numbers will take care of themselves." The private equity industry goes to great lengths to create highly complex financial models that are just thousands of numbers on a page, and that's the way they reach a conclusion about what kind of return a company will make in five years. But that's no guarantee of success if the business isn't right and the management isn't competent.

Fund I, which has now been wound up, didn't turn out very well, but the second fund has done better, and the third and fourth funds will do even better still. That's another problem with private equity. It takes many years to finally wind up the funds and the eight per cent hurdle rate is always going against you. If the partners build up some carry, as it's called, it gets eaten away by that eight per cent a year. You don't get your carry until the fund is wound up, and by then there might not be anything left to distribute.

You always hope for at least one blockbuster deal in a fund to offset the so-so deals that are inevitable and the occasional one that will flop completely. We had one excellent investment in Fund I, a company called Livingston International that is in the customs brokerage business. Livingston was very effective at consolidating an industry that until then had been dominated by small mom-and-pop operations. In Fund II, we had one or two investments that were alright, and in Fund III we're going to have one or two very good ones. The net effect is that none of the partners has really made significant money from C A I. We never paid ourselves big salaries, and Dick Schmeelk and I have been working without a salary for the past five years or so. C A I has never been a K K R or anything like that, but I have learned a lot and had the privilege to work with many talented and dedicated people. Yet I still sometimes wonder how things would have turned out if I had pursued my original idea of a boutique investment bank owned by its partners.

The C A I experience has broadened my knowledge about how Wall Street and the financial world work. One thing about C A I that I'm proud of is that when we're looking at prospective companies to buy we can tell the managers of those firms to go and talk to the managers of companies that we invested in earlier on. What they'll find is a unanimous positive opinion of C A I as an investor. We've done well by our managers. It's the old story of growing people and trusting them.

The C A I experience also taught me something about the challenges of being in business with family. Mark's involvement in C A I didn't work out ideally. Mark is a smart man but a bit shy and not a naturally gifted communicator. If you don't communicate on Wall Street, if you're not a fast talker, you don't survive. And to be honest, Mark found it a little awkward working for his dad, and I don't blame him for that. I'm not sure I would have liked working for my own father. Mark was happier and did much better after he left C A I and went off to work on his own. As for David Kauffmann, our Danish partner, he departed C A I because he wanted to live in Europe. He moved to Paris and started a successful private equity business while remaining good friends with Mark, Janice, and me.

I still haven't given up on entrepreneurship. That's where iLiv Technologies Inc. comes in. It's a software start-up founded by my son, Andrew, who is a musician, composer, and inventor. Twice in the past, Andrew asked me for financial help in starting a business, and unfortunately failure ensued. When he came to me with a third idea, I thought maybe it would be third time lucky. For me, it was clearly time for another graduation. At the age of eighty, I decided to become a venture capitalist and iLiv's sole angel investor. This has been a typically lean start-up which means that for seven years and after $2 million in funding on my part, iLiv shared offices with my investment business until recently and didn't pay any rent.

The iLiv software is designed for use in the green building industry and has an unusual philosophy behind it. It's not software that replaces any other software but instead encourages collaboration and organizes information across a broad range of subjects. One of iLiv's two customers is a California-based construction company with a reputation for using the best IT available. It calls iLiv the most intuitive software it has ever come across. I've learned that in the software business your product is never fully developed. We've been told by people in Silicon Valley that we get a mark of "A" for getting as far as we have on the basis of a $2 million investment but that we're going to need another $3 million to $4 million to get it to the next level. Our aim is to keep iLiv a family business for as long as we can. If our income begins to exceed our costs, then we'll have the choice of growing it ourselves slowly or taking in a partner and growing it faster. It's been exciting to see an idea like iLiv take flight but also somewhat of a financial strain. Behind a Japanese print hanging on the wall in my old office are two empty picture hooks. They serve as a reminder of the two paintings I had to sell to cover some of the payroll taxes iLiv owed to the government. For now, iLiv is only covering half of its cash burn out of sales, but we're still alive and the prospects remain interesting. And if we ever do make a success out of iLiv, it will give me a great deal of satisfaction.

Not surprisingly, I watched with keen interest the drama that led to the sale of Alcan to Rio Tinto in 2007. And, because Alcan was originally an offshoot of Alcoa, I suppose it was not wholly unexpected that the whole affair started with an unfriendly bid from Alcoa. It was ironic that Alcoa, the company that gave Alcan its birth, was also the company that ended up killing it! Few people were aware of how the profoundly different styles of Arthur V. Davis, the creator of Alcoa, and his younger brother Edward K. Davis, the founding C E O of Alcan, resulted in two firms with two distinctly different cultures. The likelihood of a fruitful merger was slim. At least that was my take on it when Alcoa first suggested a friendly merger in the mid-1980s when I was C E O of Alcan and Paul O'Neill ran Alcoa. His approach at that time was civilized and nonaggressive. I presume that Alcoa's approach to Alcan was different in 2007.

It was sad to see the independence of a great Canadian company disappear, but I do think there is a lot of unnecessary hysteria over foreign ownership. I have always felt that when you make an investment in another country, when you put bricks and mortar on the ground, it may belong to you in most senses, but in the extreme it doesn't. When there's a substantial investment in bricks and mortar by a foreign entity, Canadians retain a great deal of control over it because it's here, and it can't be moved. So the sale of Alcan or any other Canadian company should not provoke too much emotion.

A completely separate issue is whether there are a significant number of Canadian enterprises that are growing, adventuresome, and aggressive. Are they making investments around the world, buying up other companies, and working on the cutting edge of development? Unfortunately, we've gone through a long period when there haven't been very many of these companies. Too often, Canadian firms, led by competent, growth oriented managers, have fallen under the control of financial engineers who have sat on initiative, hated risk, and basked in the warm glow of large cash balances.

As for Alcan, I still believe it could one day end up back in Canadian hands, particularly following Rio Tinto's giant write-down on the value of its acquisition and the departure of Tom Albanese, the C E O who was the architect of the purchase. In fact, if I were younger, I'd be lining up money to buy it back. Alcan has never been a hot money maker for people, but it's been a steady earner over the years and could be an excellent investment for Canadian pension funds.

My new life after graduation from Alcan also gave me more time to pursue another career of sorts, one in the nonprofit world. While at Alcan, I had been on various boards including McGill University, the Montreal Symphony Orchestra, and the Business Council on National Issues, but, because of my day job, I wasn't able to devote much time to outside organizations. That changed with retirement ... er, graduation.

When it came to charitable giving, I believed that, from Alcan's viewpoint, small was beautiful. I found that the company could do more good by responding on short notice to a plea for $10,000 from the McGill Chamber Orchestra or another small charity than by donating $1 million to a well-established charity. We would make large contributions at times, as we did when we backed establishment of the Alcan Study Centre at the Canadian Centre for Architecture, but, in general, I believed we would get more bang for our buck by supporting small, volunteer-supported organizations. I was considered a soft touch when it came to these kinds of appeals, especially when they came from people like Hollis Marden.

Hollis was an American who worked for years as an executive at Domtar. When he retired, Hollis took on the leadership of two venerable Montreal charitable institutions, the Queen Elizabeth Hospital and the Mackay Centre for Deaf and Crippled Children. He rented an office in the Sun Life Building and dedicated himself to overseeing these philanthropic endeavours. Hollis was a fabulous money raiser. He'd call me on a Wednesday and tell me, "David, we have a real problem moving our students around town. They're handicapped and need special vehicles. And you know what? There's a bus for sale in Ohio that suits our needs perfectly." I'd say to him, "Would $10,000 help?" And Hollis would respond, "Oh, fantastic! You're great!" A day later, Hollis would call me again and say, "David, it's not quite enough. I need a bit more cash to buy the bus." And, inevitably, I would add to the original pledge.

Sometimes, people's motivations for giving can be a bit obscure. One day, as I was walking to work with Hollis, he asked me whether I knew a man named Sydenham B. Lindsay. I said I thought that that there was a Protestant minister by that name who had lived on McTavish Street when my family was on Peel Street. It turns out that Rev. Lindsay was a regular contributor to the Queen Elizabeth Hospital, usually in small amounts. He would send over cheques of $19.61 or $25.32 that he endorsed to the hospital. Hollis explained, "I always write to him and thank him when one of his cheques arrives, and I always ask him to drop by the hospital and meet the doctors and nurses and see what we are doing with his money. And he never comes. The other day I got to my office at the Queen Elizabeth Hospital and there on my desk was a cheque for $10,000 signed by Sydenham B. Lindsay. This time, I was determined to get the pastor over to the hospital to thank him for his generosity. So I called, and his son answered. When I explained that we wanted to thank his father for his generous gift, the son responded that it must be a misunderstanding because his father didn't have the means to make $10,000 donations. But he said there was another Sydenham B. Lindsay in Montreal who worked on St James Street in the financial business who might be the donor." Hollis got the phone number for the second Mr Lindsay and called him with a thank you and an invitation to visit the hospital. "Mr Marden, I don't give a damn what you do with that money," he responded. "I'm not in the least bit interested." Hollis asked him why he had given such a big donation if he really didn't care what happened to it. Mr Lindsay responded, "Mr Marden, any institution in Montreal that has the guts to name itself after Queen Elizabeth gets $10,000 from me."

While still at Alcan, I was asked to help out Miss Edgar's and Miss Cramp's School for Girls, an independent school which both Mary and Diane attended. In the early 1960s, the school ran into a crisis when Montreal Mayor Jean Drapeau did a deal allowing a developer to build an apartment building on the site of the school on Côte-des-Neiges Road. The school had been renting an old house that was to be torn down to make way for the development, and, with little time to spare, we had to find alternative accommodations. I was approached by Hazel Harrington, a board member who had been asked to lead the relocation effort but had only agreed to do so if she could get the help of a businessman such as myself. During the next eight months, Hazel and I worked like dogs, finding a site and building a facility to accommodate the students. We found a piece of land on Mount Pleasant Avenue, a quiet street in Westmount that would be a big improvement on the old site, which in any case had too much traffic. I suggested that we also buy the rambling house just above the new site and locate the kindergarten and grade one girls there. I figured the smaller girls would feel more comfortable in a house than in an institutional building. I didn't get my choice of architect for the new building because the board had already hired one, but he ended up doing a very good job.

Independent schools became a kind of calling for me. I served on the board of Selwyn House and later became its chairman at a time when the headmaster was a man named Dr Speirs. He had taught me when I was a student at Lower Canada College in 1939 and eventually moved to Selwyn House where he was appointed headmaster. When Dr Speirs retired after twenty-five years heading the school, I asked him what the secret of his success was. He had a way of looking skyward before he answered a question. He lifted his head, thought a moment, and said, "Boys first, teachers second, parents third." A very sound approach to running any school.

Volunteer boards are the most difficult boards to manage. Bill Bowen, a fellow director on the American Express board, once passed me a note that said, "Good intentions randomize behaviour!" Nowhere does that apply more than with volunteer, non-profit boards! Nobody is being paid a penny, but everybody has a surplus of good intentions, and some see their board membership as a license to run wild. It's amazing how a well-intentioned individual can be named to a hospital board, suddenly feel personally responsible for everything that's going on in the place, and believe it's up to them to correct the situation when an orderly has been impolite to a patient or when they hear of some person who had to wait a few hours to be treated in the emergency room.

In the late 1990s, Bernard Shapiro, McGill's principal, approached me at least twice to become chair of the McGill University Health Centre (MUHC), which had been formed from the consolidation of five historic institutions including the Royal Victoria Hospital, the Montreal General Hospital, the Montreal Chest Institute, the Montreal Children's Hospital, and the Montreal Neurological Institute and Hospital. Hospitals are not institutions normally designed to merge, what with their cherished histories, their individual boards, and their fiefdoms of doctors and administrators, yet here we had a voluntary merger of five hospitals. They decided to merge in 1994, and Hugh Scott was the first director general of the combined hospital. People don't always give him a lot of credit, but he managed to get from five chief surgeons down to one, five chief nurses down to one, etc., which as you can imagine wasn't easy. What remains extraordinary is that it was all voluntary. One of the big differences between the McGill hospital and the CHUM, the merger of the big Montreal francophone hospitals that formed University of Montreal Hospital Centre, is that the government had to force the University of Montreal hospitals to merge. That shotgun marriage remains problematic to this day.

The director general of the Montreal Children's Hospital at the time of the merger was Dr Nicolas Steinmetz, and, with typical German logic, he said that it made no sense to have five McGill-affiliated hospitals, six if you include the Jewish General Hospital, all on different sites with facilities in urgent need of modernization. He felt that they should be combined into one hospital and should all be on one site. When the merger later became so difficult I sometimes wondered why they had ever voluntarily merged. The cultural divide was great. One of Mary's best friends was married to a doctor at the Montreal General, and she used to refer to the Royal Victoria, known popularly as the Royal Vic, as "that other hospital." When the merger took place, it turned out that most of the individuals chosen for the senior surgical and medical positions came from the Royal Vic. It just worked out that way, but it exacerbated the feeling at the Montreal General that they were being taken over by the Royal Vic. As for the Children's Hospital, the sentiment among many there was that the people who ran the adult hospitals didn't understand what pediatric medicine was all about, and they believed that they could raise their own money and didn't need help from anybody else. There's still a bit of a separatist movement at the Children's Hospital that is fed by a recurring sense that the hospital's very existence is under threat. Every now and again some civil servant in Quebec City will say that Montreal does not need two pediatric hospitals and that we should close the Montreal Children's Hospital and just retain Sainte-Justine Hospital. Utter nonsense.

Once the new McGill hospital is completed, attention will turn to the future of the old Royal Victoria Hospital, a collection of nineteenth century stone buildings built in the Scottish baronial style on the flanks of Mount Royal. My suggestion would be to gut the buildings, leave the walls standing, and let the air blow through for six months to get rid of more than a century of germs. But anybody who thinks these architectural gems will be converted to luxury condominiums will be disappointed. Donald Smith and George Stephen, the Canadian Pacific Railway tycoons who financed the original construction of the Royal Vic, wisely stipulated that if the original buildings were no longer used for the health and welfare of Montrealers, their ownership would revert to their heirs and descendants. Knowing that a new hospital was being built, these descendants would occasionally contact us from all over the world, and ask us what our plans were for the future of the Royal Vic, clearly not wanting to miss out on their inheritance if the old buildings were ultimately sold as part of a commercial venture. My view is that McGill should use the original hospital buildings for medical research while the later additions should be converted into new student residences, which McGill badly needs.

A major challenge in building the new hospital campus was to convince the Shriners to relocate its long-established Montreal hospital from Cedar Avenue to the new site and to not simply move it elsewhere in Canada. The hospital, though small, is the only such facility the Shriners run in Canada and does highly specialized pediatric orthopedic research in conjunction with McGill. They not only look after children from Quebec, Ontario, and the Maritimes but also from the northern US states as well. The day after I became chairman of the M U H C, Richard Cruess, who was the Dean of Medicine at McGill at the time, told me that if there's one thing I had to do in my new job, it was keep the Shriners in Montreal. McGill didn't want to lose the Shriners but neither did the city nor the province want to see it leave. It turned out to be a valuable weapon for the M U H C. The new hospital is being built on the site of an old Canadian Pacific train yard at the Glen in lower Westmount that needed a major environmental cleanup before construction could begin. At one point, the government wouldn't even let us move forward and clean up the land, arguing that we had to wait for the University of Montreal hospital project to move forward. We went directly to Premier Jean Charest and told him that if the McGill hospital didn't get built soon the Shriners would simply move their facility to London, Ontario or to Ottawa. The cleanup went ahead, construction of the complex is well underway, and the new hospital is set to open in early 2015.

Premier Charest, Mayor Tremblay, and the hospital leadership actually attended Shriners conventions in Florida and in Baltimore to close the deal. What made the Montreal case more challenging is the fact that the Shriners had hardly any members in Quebec. During the lobbying efforts, I had some dealings with Gene Bracewell, the Imperial Treasurer of the Shriners, who was from Atlanta and no friend of the Montreal position. The first time he came to town after I became chairman, I took him to lunch at the Mount Royal Club. "I was eighteen years old when I met my wife," he told me in his Georgia drawl. "And when we were about to get married, her father lined the two of us up and said, 'Bracewell, if you ever cheat on my daughter, I'll kill you,' and he looked at his daughter and said, 'And if you ever come home for any reason other than he's cheatin' on you, I'll lock the door.'" Real southern stuff. In the end, the Shriners decided that they would build at the

Glen, raising their own money for a six-storey, $127 million hospital that will open a year later than the rest of the new facility.

Our original idea was to build the complete new hospital on the Glen site and close the Montreal General, which dates from the 1950s, as well as the ancient facilities at the Royal Victoria. But the government didn't like that option, and I must admit that they were partly right, so the decision was made to keep the Montreal General buildings on the slopes of Mount Royal. We managed to turn the decision to keep operating on two sites into an advantage by putting elective medicine at the new hospital while leaving emergency medicine at the Montreal General. We figured that when you have both elective and emergency medicine on the same site, elective surgery always gets bumped in favour of an emergency.

One of the reasons I was originally reluctant to take the job of MUHC chairman is that I'm not a good fundraiser, and I knew that the hospital needed to raise a huge amount of money for its "Best Care for Life" campaign. I simply don't have the knack for hitting people up for money. Knowing my own shortcomings, I was fortunate enough to convince John Rae of Power Corp, who is a superb fundraiser, to head the campaign. He's done a marvellous job. The original goal was $328 million, and John has stuck with it for six or seven years, and so far he has raised about $300 million out of that total.

In 2007, the government decreed that hospital boards were to be reelected for three-year terms. I had been chairman for seven years. I said that I was prepared to carry on but maybe not for another three years, knowing that there are always people on a volunteer board who would like to take over. The machinery went into motion, and one day a couple of members of the board came by to see me and asked if I would be ready to step aside and allow David Angus to become chairman. It was time for another graduation. I stepped down willingly, but I still follow the course of events at the MUHC closely and am excited at the prospect of the new hospital finally coming to fruition after so many years of patience and hard work.

I look back at my seven years as chairman of the M U H C with a mixture of pride and regret. Pride due to the care that will be provided at the Glen and Mountain sites of the new hospital and pride in the doctors, nurses and administrators responsible for that care. Regret that the tension between what I call Old Quebec and New Quebec led to delays and massive cost escalations and removed the hospital board from any say in who, how, and with what architectural style the project would be carried out. As the charming and forceful Quebec finance minister told me in the middle of my tenure as chairman, "David, over my dead body will we let you build the new hospital the way you want to." But I feel warm and grateful when I contemplate the care that Montrealers will receive at the new M U H C hospital in the future.

It has now been more than twenty years since my graduation from Alcan and my second career at C A I began. Admittedly, C A I is no longer taking the same amount of my time as it once did and the day-to-day running of the business has shifted to a new generation and away from Dick Schmeelk and me. That is the way it should be. We have always wanted C A I to become a sustainable business for the long run.

Much of the focus of my business life is now with iLiv, not just as an investor, but also as a provider of, hopefully, sage advice. In my 80s, I've learned to enjoy the occasional trip to Silicon Valley and to understand a way of doing business that's light years away from my early days of selling carloads of aluminum to independent fabricators in small-town Pennsylvania. But it's also time for iLiv to start flying on its own, so its cohabitation arrangement with C A I has come to an end, and they have moved to their own premises. After a long sojourn in the old greystone house on Drummond Street, Janice and I have moved across the street to a more modest yet comfortable office in a modern apartment building a few steps up the hill and just a couple of blocks from where I grew up. It was time for a new graduation.

I still look at every day as a remarkable gift offering so much to enjoy and get pleasure from, whether it's in the form of a spirited doubles match on the tennis court, the opportunity of seeing a granddaughter acting her heart out in a university production, or the sight of the sun sparkle on the snow of a frozen Lake Manitou. I believe it was Albert Einstein who once remarked, "There are only two ways to live your life. One is as though nothing is a miracle. The other is as though everything is a miracle." I choose the latter.